The Age of Optimal Health

Revised and Updated

A Comprehensive Guide for Men Over 50 to Maintain an Active Lifestyle, Ensure Proper Nutrition, and Take Preventative Measures

By Surleigh Tara

ISBN: 979-8-9887665-0-6

"As an airline pilot in my 50s, I highly recommend **The Age of Optimal Health** for its comprehensive approach to maintaining peak performance as we age. The book's emphasis on nutrition and exercise resonated with me, as it highlighted the importance of fueling our bodies properly and staying physically active to meet the demands of our profession. With practical exercises for maintaining flexibility and balance and tips for managing hormonal changes, this book offers a roadmap to optimal health, especially for those who sit for hours on end, whether in the cockpit or behind a desk. I've been flying for over 30 years and have read numerous books on health and well-being, but I have found many suggestions either contradict each other or are difficult to follow due to my busy schedule. I highly recommend this book for anyone seeking practical tips to offset the mental and physical challenges as we age."

Johnny Aliksa Duffy
Airline Pilot

*"**The Age of Optimal Health** by Surleigh Tara is a must-read for men over 50 seeking to enhance their well-being. With a wealth of knowledge of exercise, nutrition, mental health, and financial planning, Surleigh provides practical advice alongside personal anecdotes that make the book relevant and engaging. The book offers valuable insights and actionable steps for achieving lifelong vitality."*

Maged Y. Gerges, M.ED., AET
Director of Culinary Excellence
Company Executive Chef | TG Tasty
Foods INC

"The author approaches turning 50 as a critical milestone for males to positively shape their life trajectories on multiple fronts. The book highlights many of the prevailing challenges that men in this age group face and outlines simple preventative strategies and practical disciplines to help promote healthier, more active lifestyles! It even ventures into social, mental, and financial health issues to prove a comprehensive blueprint that all men can easily follow in this significant season! It's like having a life coach wrapped up in a captivating book! Well worth the read."

Sanjeev Nandakumaran, MD
Family Medicine Physician Leader,
Southern California Permanente
Medical Group

Medical Disclaimer

The information presented in this book, *The Age of Optimal Health: A Comprehensive Guide for Men Over 50 to Maintain an Active Lifestyle, Ensure Proper Nutrition, and Take Preventative Measures*, authored by Surleigh Tara, is for informational purposes only.

The content provided in this book is not intended to be a substitute for professional medical advice, diagnosis, or treatment. Always seek the advice of your physician or other qualified health provider with any questions you may have regarding a medical condition. Never disregard professional medical advice or delay seeking it because of something you have read in this book.

The author and publisher of this book have made reasonable efforts to ensure that the information provided is accurate and up to date at the time of publication. However, medical knowledge constantly evolves, and new research may emerge that could change the data presented. Therefore, the author and publisher do not guarantee the accuracy, completeness, or timeliness of the information contained within this book. The author and publisher of this book are not liable for any losses, injuries, or damages arising from using the information provided. The reader should consult a healthcare professional before significantly changing their diet, exercise routine, or lifestyle.

The mention of specific products, services, or organizations within this book does not imply endorsement by the author or publisher. Including such information is purely for illustrative purposes and does not constitute a recommendation.

The responsibility for interpreting and using the information presented in this book lies solely with the reader. The author and publisher disclaim any liability or responsibility for any adverse effects arising from using or applying the information contained herein.

By reading this book, you acknowledge that you have read and understood this medical disclaimer. You agree to release the author, publisher, and any associated individuals from any liability or responsibility for any claims, damages, or injuries arising from using or applying the information provided in this book.

Always consult a qualified healthcare professional for any personalized medical advice and recommendations.

Dedication

This book is dedicated with my gratitude and love to all of you and all men over 50 striving for optimal health and well-being. May God richly bless all of you reading this book, and may it help you significantly on your journey!

Thank you for allowing me to be a part of your life's story. Together, we will reach new heights! God bless you all! I thank you from the bottom of my heart. May the Lord bless and keep you always!

Acknowledgment

I thank the Almighty God for granting me the opportunity and courage to write this book.

First and foremost, I am eternally grateful to my family, who have been a constant source of love, support, and inspiration. To my three brothers and their wives, Palokoa (*fmr.* USMC) and Jocelin, Tara and Ilis, and Burleigh (*ret.* US Army) and Sepe (*fmr.* US Army), thank you for always standing by my side and providing unwavering encouragement throughout this endeavor. Your presence and encouragement have meant the world to me. I would also like to acknowledge my mother, Niokong Charley Tara, who is still with us and in the loving memory of my late father, Yukiwo Nemia Tara. Their love and guidance have shaped me into the person I am today, and I carry their memories with me in every word I write.

I am deeply grateful to my family, especially my wife, Eleanor, and our children, Trevor, Vanessa, Chelsea, and Zachariah, for their unwavering love and support. I sincerely appreciate everyone who has contributed to the launch of my book. Ako Harper from Garage Warrior, thank you so much for allowing me to use your photo for the cover; it truly encapsulates my story.

A special mention goes out to Karnim Judah and MSgt RunnyMoky Kilafwasru (USAF) for their devoted proofreading, which helped bring the manuscript to life. My ministry partners, Pastor Sato Suka, Pastor Lawrence Yinolang (*fmr.* USMC), Pastor Charles Hartman, Pastor Arnold Marcus (*ret. LtCol,* US Army), Pastor Herbert Sigrah, Dcn. Driskell Jack, Dcn. McGill Tolenna, Mr. Lipan Welly (*ret.* US Army), Mr. Frank Alokoa, and my sister Dcnse. Hanna Alokoa - your guidance and feedback were essential for a successful launch. The Pasifika Publishing Facebook group provided invaluable insight as well.

The collaboration between Dr. Sanjeev Nandakumaran, MD, and Mr. Kelroy Kohatsu has resulted in a powerful resource that empowers readers to take control of their overall health and financial well-being. The expertise of Dr. Nandakumaran has been invaluable in revising "The Age of Optimal Health," infusing it with personal insights and practical wisdom. His guidance on sharing experiences has made the content more relatable and impactful, inspiring readers to act toward their optimal health. Meanwhile, Mr. Kohatsu's insights on the financial aspects of indexing strategy have shed invaluable light on emerging trends in the financial industry. Together, these two experts have created an engaging and informative resource that informs and inspires readers to take charge of their physical and financial well-being.

Finally, my sincere gratitude goes to all of you, the readers, who have taken the time to read my book. I am humbled and honored. May you all be blessed!

About the Author

Surleigh Tara is the Founder and CEO of Kahs in Kol, Inc. (also known as Pasifika United), a non-profit ministry dedicated to empowering leaders in growing Pacific Island communities with the tools they need to reach out to their communities with the Gospel. Surleigh earned his master's in divinity from Azusa Pacific University and is pursuing a Doctor of Philosophy (Ph.D.) in Bible Exposition at Liberty University, where they train students to become "Champions for Christ." Surleigh has experienced a life-changing transition- from a successful, fulfilling career in the Information Technology field to leading a full-time nonprofit ministry. With over 18 years of experience in IT, he spent 13 years at Azusa Pacific University (APU), where he rose to the position of Business Enterprise Systems Analyst. His decision to pursue full-time ministry was driven by a deep passion to provide spiritual guidance and support for those struggling with faith. His nonprofit organization has already achieved a great deal in offering comfort and hope through Jesus Christ. His journey from the corporate world to ministry has been inspiring, and he continues to make a meaningful impact on people's lives.

Surleigh is married to Eleanor Marcus Tara and is the father of four children — Trevor, Vanessa, Chelsea, and Zachariah. His family is incredibly thankful for the love and guidance that God has provided them, allowing Surleigh to live out his calling with Kahs in Kol, Inc. His ministry is for everyone, and his dedication to its cause brings him great joy in knowing he can share the love of Jesus with those who need it most.

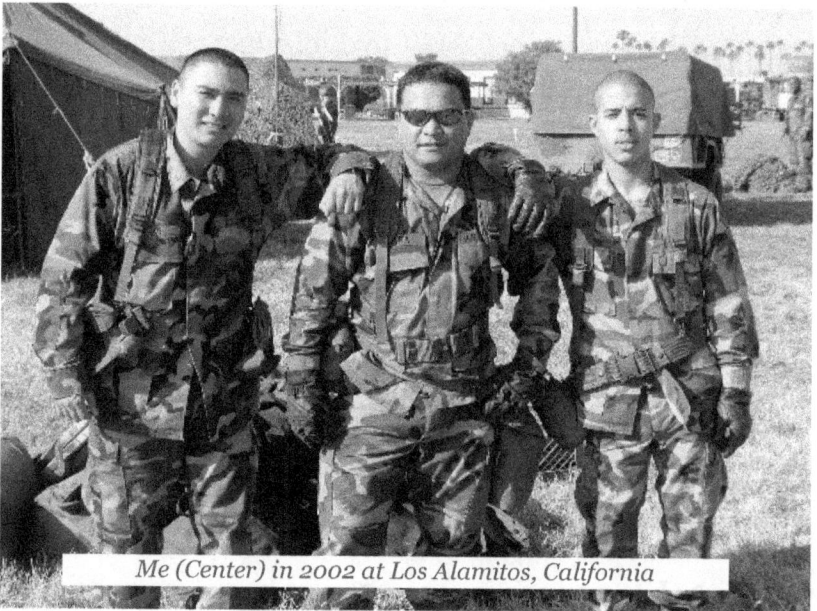

Me (Center) in 2002 at Los Alamitos, California

Surleigh was once in excellent physical condition as a U.S. military veteran until a few years after his honorable discharge. After several years of encountering various illnesses and numerous efforts to regain optimal health, he ultimately stumbled upon a solution that propelled him to complete wellness and inspired him to write this book. His persistence and hard work eventually led to the publication of this book, *The Age of Optimal Health,* in which he details the journey that led to his recovery. Surleigh is a true testament to the power of faith and commitment and continues to use this to inspire those around him. He hopes to continue his ministry work with Kahs in Kol until he retires, inspiring others around the globe through his work and dedication.

Surleigh firmly believes that everyone has the potential to live an abundant life and achieve great things if only they are willing to put in the hard work and dedication it takes to make that happen. By sharing his story, he hopes to show people how faith, commitment, and perseverance are necessary for optimal health and wellness.

Contents

Introduction

"Age is not lost youth but a new stage of opportunity and strength."

-Betty Friedan

We all know that staying nutritious and active is one of the most satisfactory ways to keep our bodies healthy. But do you understand it can also improve your well-being and quality of life?

The trick to staying healthy and active at all life stages is finding something you enjoy doing. For some, that means having a companion to exercise with. It doesn't matter whether you're going to the jogging track or gym, walking around the block, dancing along to an aerobics DVD in a private room, or going out for a quiet bike ride—get moving.

Finding your workout style can be formidable; it can mix it up occasionally. You may want to try something new. Some unique strategies are described in the book to engage and hook people who wish to get active and stay active. No matter what age you are, the truth is that your body slowly loses its energy, strength, stamina, and ability to function appropriately without regular activity. It's like the old saying:

"You don't stop moving from growing old; you grow old from stopping movements."

Exercise increases muscle power, increasing your capacity to do other physical activities. It's true—60 is the new 50—but only if you're healthy. People who are physically or mentally active live about seven to ten years longer than those who are not active and are obese. The noteworthy part is that those additional years are generally healthier! Staying active helps delay or avoid chronic illnesses and diseases associated with aging. Thus, active adults increase their quality of life and independence even as they age.

The book *The Age of Optimal Health: A Comprehensive Guide for Men Over 50 to Maintain an Active Lifestyle, Ensure Proper Nutrition, and Take Preventative Measures* provides a comprehensive overview of how men over 50 can maintain optimal health and well-being. It covers benefits and challenges, obesity and nutrition, promoting an active lifestyle, preventative measures, erectile dysfunction, mental health, social health, and financial health to give readers practical advice on leading a balanced life. With its wide range of information, this book is an invaluable resource for men entering the prime of adulthood.

Most people over the age of 50 tend to overlook their health. Many reasons compelled me to write this book, such as the need for more information or the misbelief that health and well-being can be taken care of later in life. Many Christian men are also in this same difficulty. With this book, I hope to give people the tools and knowledge to take charge of their health and lead fulfilling lives. This book will provide practical strategies for physical fitness, nutrition, preventive health screenings, and mental health. It will also include advice on coping with the effects of the COVID-19 pandemic on mental health and Christian practices that can help promote optimal health. Ultimately, this book aims to empower men to live their best lives and reach their full potential.

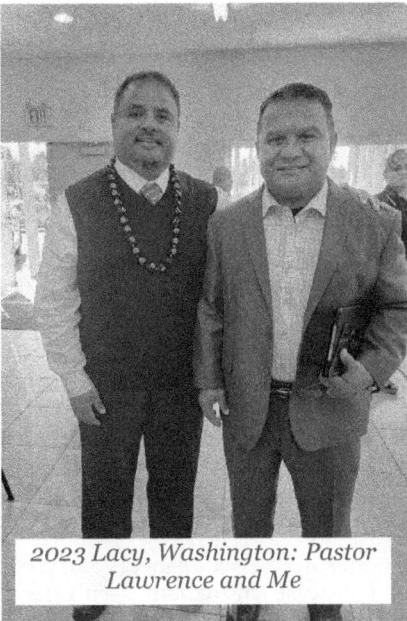

2023 Lacy, Washington: Pastor Lawrence and Me

As men enter the 50th year of their lives, it is essential to promote an active lifestyle through regular exercise, proper nutrition, and preventative screenings such as prostate exams to ensure optimal physical and mental health. These recommendations should begin early on and continue throughout all stages of life, allowing for both short-term and long-term benefits.

Follow a healthy lifestyle by taking a low-fat diet and exercising daily. Both things cannot be overlooked at any stage of life, especially in old age, where fats and carbohydrates deposit quickly into the body, leading to diabetes, hypercholesterolemia, and many other cardiovascular diseases.[1] In recent decades, many studies have proved that dietary patterns and junk food intake affect lifestyle.

A good and balanced diet bestows well-being and longevity to a person. People who follow active lifestyles sustain happy relationships, heed spiritual needs, and reduce stress levels.

When considering diet after age 50, studies and research support the common wisdom of eating a well-balanced diet low in fat and high in fresh fruits and vegetables. Achieving or maintaining a healthy weight is especially necessary at this age and can contribute to a longer life.

According to the American Heart Association's Nutrition Committee, maintaining a healthy body weight, eating low-

---

[1] Paquette M, Bernard S, Ruel I, Blank DW, Genest J, Baass A. Diabetes is associated with an increased risk of cardiovascular disease in patients with familial hypercholesterolemia. J Clin Lipidol. 2019 Jan–Feb;13(1):123-128. doi: 10.1016/j.jacl.2018.09.008. Epub 2018 Sep 17. PMID: 30318454.

carb and low-fat foods, exercising regularly, avoiding tobacco, and avoiding alcohol are crucial to heart health.[2] These recommendations are significant since cardiovascular and heart diseases are among the most common causes of demise for people over 50.

Living a healthy lifestyle is essential for making the most out of our lives, but there is no one-size-fits-all solution. When asking 50 people about their take on a healthy lifestyle, you will get 50 different answers. There are no hard and fast rules to define a healthy lifestyle. Staying active and joyful is the key to living healthy, and it varies from person to person. For some, regular exercise like jogging or running, eating fast food once a week, and spending quality time with loved ones may be the answer. For others, pushing themselves to run a marathon, strict fasting or keto diets, and abstaining from alcohol may be the ideal health regime. There is no right or wrong way of pursuing a healthy lifestyle. What matters is choosing the path that aligns with our needs and aspirations. We must follow our hearts and seek the best healthy lifestyle for us.

Before continuing, let me inject relevant geographical

---

[2] (2023), Heart Attack and Stroke Symptoms, American Heart Association, Retrieve from https://www.heart.org/en/news/2019/03/25/what-kind-of-diet-helps-heart-health.

information about my origin. In the Pacific Ocean are four major groups of islands. They are as follows: Indonesia, Melanesia, Micronesia, and Polynesia. The Federated States of Micronesia (FSM) is a sovereign nation in the Micronesia region. The FSM, too, has four groups of islands that are categorized as states. The four states are Chuuk, Kosrae, Pohnpei, and Yap. The capital city of FSM is Palikir, on Pohnpei's island.

Growing up in the Micronesia region on Kosrae Island, I was fortunate to be surrounded by abundant natural food sources, particularly from the ocean. However, as a young man, I succumbed to societal pressures to eat processed foods imported from outside sources. Looking back, I realize this was a mistake and that the allure of being seen as more advanced and modern wasn't worth the cost. Unfortunately, many people in the Pacific Islands have also given up their traditional ways of life and have replaced them with non-perishable canned foods imported from elsewhere. We must understand the implications of our choice to consume imported foods over locally sourced ones and make a concerted effort to preserve our cultural and natural heritage. I am passionate about promoting healthy and sustainable living in the Pacific Islands. We should all prioritize what's best for our environment and communities.

A healthy lifestyle can help you feel happy, decrease the risk of some dangerous diseases, increase your lifespan, save money, and benefit the environment. Your remodeled version of a healthy lifestyle is whatever you define it to be. There's nothing in life you must or must not do to be healthy. Identify what makes you feel good and brings you the most distinguished joy. Then, start with something small when you make some amendments or changes in your life. You're more likely to see success this way, and small wins will snowball into more significant benefits.

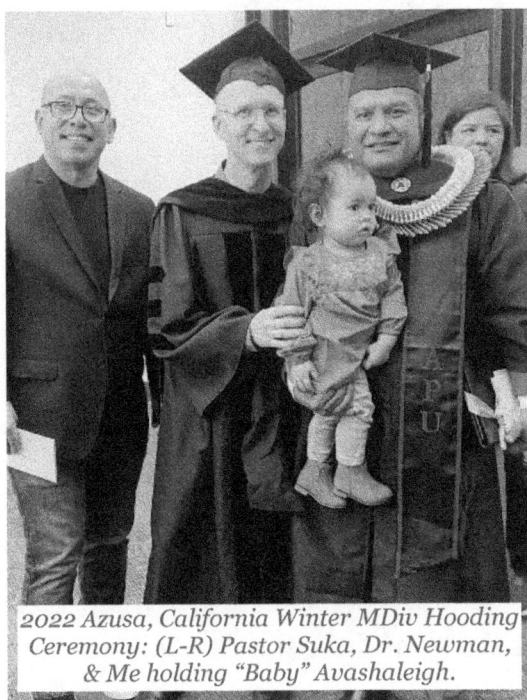

2022 Azusa, California Winter MDiv Hooding Ceremony: (L-R) Pastor Suka, Dr. Newman, & Me holding "Baby" Avashaleigh.

Growing older doesn't mean giving up your morning run. It was a common belief when people thought running could wreck their knees. However, new studies and research suggest it can strengthen the knees and core by strengthening the muscles that protect them. And it doesn't raise your risk of joint problems or arthritis. If you have arthritis or damaged joints, running could be too much. But you can still benefit from exercise. Low-impact activities like walking or biking can help strengthen muscles, support joints, and lessen pain.

Amaze yourself!

Instead of sticking with what's comfortable and familiar, tackle something new. For example, I started farming and raising livestock several months before writing this book. This new way keeps me busy; whether it be pulling out weeds, trimming trees in my orchard, feeding and moving my cows, pigs, goats, turkeys, or chickens, or performing daily routines like cleaning pens and coops; these new tasks give me a unique perspective of appreciating life.

There are other options, like going to out-of-the-ordinary places. Try to make new friends at the different sites you visit. Try to learn some musical instrument or any new language. Unique and new experiences will build new pathways in your brain, keeping your mind healthy as you age. All these things help you be healthy inside and out. They'll also expand your options for finding excitement and happiness. The older people get, the more satisfied and content they are. People in their 70s report being more confident than people in their

60s.[3] So, try to look forward to the future optimistically and innovatively instead of thinking most of your time has passed away because right now could be a time of great happiness and inner satisfaction.

Having spent over 15 years in the ministry, I deeply understand offering spiritual guidance and hope through Jesus Christ. Many men in their prime years work around the clock to create wealth while neglecting the care that the body needs. As a result, in later years, the broken body needs repairing. Instead of enjoying the money earned, it is utilized to fix the damaged body. The last resort to preserve health when all else fails is returning to the Creator of all creations.

Without proper health, it is impossible to serve God actively. There may be other indirect ways, but not typical ways to be physically present. This does not mean an unhealthy person cannot serve God. God is a loving God who always makes a way when there is a will.

The launch of this book was initially intended for the people of Kosrae (where I am from), especially those like me, who were at one point in their lives on the verge of facing health issues. The more I researched the topic, I discovered that it

---

[3] This is the Exact Age When the Average Person Is Most Confident, The Healthy, Retrieved from: https://www.thehealthy.com/mental-health/self-care/age-when-average-person-most-confident/

9

was not only a Kosraean problem but more of a Micronesia regional issue. Then, I looked further into it to learn that it was not only a Micronesian issue but a Pacific Islander health concern. More research done now proves that this is a global problem.

As a U.S. military veteran, I understand the importance of physical and spiritual health and wellness from first-hand experience. After my enlistment, my health started deteriorating because of my addictions to tobacco products and alcohol. I didn't care too much about the type of food I was eating, nor did I make time to have a physical check-up with my doctor. I can't remember whether I had a doctor or not.

Although I was in excellent condition during my service, my exposure to illnesses and experiences recovering from illnesses gave me insight into the challenges of achieving true wellness. Through faith and dedication, I overcame my struggles and, since then, have been helping many others in similar circumstances. With this knowledge and experience, I am uniquely qualified to write *The Age of Optimal Health*. I am passionate about helping people from all walks of life achieve optimal health and live their best lives. The knowledge I have gained through this journey has allowed me to share my insights with others and help them begin their journey toward optimal health. With my experience, I can comprehensively look at the many aspects of health and wellness, from physical to mental and spiritual well-being. With this book, I aim to give readers an accurate, honest, and reliable look at the steps necessary to achieve optimal health and share what I have experienced in my journey.

The ideas and concepts in the book will serve a solid purpose for improving health patterns in people over 50. Being physically active is not solely what good health means. This also includes mental and emotional fitness levels, meaning the human body must live healthily inside and out. It should be part of everyone's lifestyle, but as a person ages, he is likely to suffer more due to a compromised immune system or other co-morbidities. Hence, adopting a healthy lifestyle at all ages and stages of life is essential.

Life is amazing. Anything that dims your spirit toward accomplishing your goal should be eradicated. Whenever you feel any dip in your motivation, you can choose this book and value your body, soul, and mind, as it will groom you to live a beautiful life. Remove all unhealthy and tempting things that distract you from your goal of living the best life. The aim is to help a maximum number of people over 50 who live inactive and sedentary lifestyles. Hence, they know all the tips, techniques, and tricks to stay healthy and fit without worrying about age. This book has been written in a rousing style, covering all mental and physical health considerations for people over 50 and providing them with information in an inspirational way that could help them relive every single moment of their lives.

Chapter 1: Benefits and Challenges

"The Truth Is, the Harder You Fight, the Sweeter Are the Rewards in the End."

~Mary Kom

Stress Management:

No matter where you come from or where you live, you must have experienced or may still be experiencing stress.

It may have several underlying issues, including something going wrong in your personal or professional life. Sometimes, people experience a significant amount of stress when they face financial problems.

Our bodies tend to respond to stress in specific ways to protect ourselves. It switches to protective and survival mode when we face extreme pressure, such as being faced with a predator or lost in the middle of nowhere. However, such events aren't expected to occur in our lives, but that does not take away the stress we face in this fast-moving, chaotic world around us.

The kind of stress that we experience in our daily lives is

related to our personal and professional lives. Some people may face pressure because their day started on a sour note. What accelerates that stress is when they end up having numerous deadlines and a significant workload. Financial management can also be an issue for many people, causing them stress regarding paying their bills, saving for their future, or investing for retirement. Our minds and bodies react to this stress as fighters because we see it as a threat. However, as common as anxiety is, managing it before it starts gripping our minds and actions is in our hands.

We should consider noticing how our body reacts to stress. It usually happens when we experience something we perceive as a threat to ourselves.

For example, you are late for work, and your car has broken down. You've tried everything possible to start your car's engine but failed. You are already late, and knowing this has already triggered your stress. Now, one option is to take the subway to work. You rush to take your belongings from the car and reach the station.

As you wait for the train to arrive, you see a homeless guy coming to where you are standing. You try to ignore the eye contact and hope he passes you, but your brain is sending signals to be cautious of the guy. The guy stands right next to you, which makes you more uncomfortable. At this moment, the hypothalamus—a small part of your brain's base—starts alarming your body to be in fight or flight mode. Your body utilizes a combination of nerves and the hormonal signals they send, which prompt your adrenal glands to release hormones such as cortisol and adrenaline. When you experience this adrenaline rush, your heartbeat will increase, increasing your blood pressure and energy supplies. The stress hormone that increases the glucose level in your bloodstream is cortisol. It also enhances the brain's glucose utilization, multiplying the repaired tissue substances.

Cortisol tends to introduce alterations to the functionality of a human's immune system. It causes severe impacts on a person's digestive, growth, and reproductive systems. It triggers a natural alarm that also affects the parts of the brain that regulate a person's mood, motivation, and paranoia. Cortisol is also known to have severe side effects on a person, and it may also cause a person to react in a manner not required during a flight-or-fight incident.

Some people still experience the side effects even after they've experienced a stressful event in their lives. Although a person's heart rate and hormones return to normal when they feel safe and not under any threat, they will always keep a person's stressors activated, which can be triggered by something reminding them of their past traumatic experiences. These stressors can also activate due to minor stressful situations, including arguing with someone or having a hectic day at work.

When you experience a prolonged stress response, system activation can expose you to the threat of severe bodily dysfunctions. It may cause numerous health issues that may go undetected if not given proper attention. These health risks include anxiety, migraines, strain and muscle pain, fatigue, cardiovascular dysfunctions, strokes, insomnia, obesity, digestive issues, depression, ADHD, and dementia.

Learning to control stress before it starts controlling you physically, psychologically, and emotionally is imperative. It would be best to consider that before reaching out to someone for help when you are stressed; they may not give you the solution you seek. Stress is subjective from person to person based on their experiences in life. You may be stressed because of something the other person may consider typical. Under any circumstances, you should avoid getting discouraged by any critical advice someone may give you. It would be best never to neglect your stress and the elements causing it, i.e., your stressors. How we react to our stress elements is unique and different from others. Our response to specific stressors may be different from that of our friends or family members experiencing the same thing. They may have a contrasting impact of their stressful events on them than us. We should work on dealing with our stress more healthily. We can't change or alter our situations, but we can always take control of how we react to situations causing us stress. If we learn how to manage and control the impact our stressful events have on us, we can unlock the potential of healthy living.

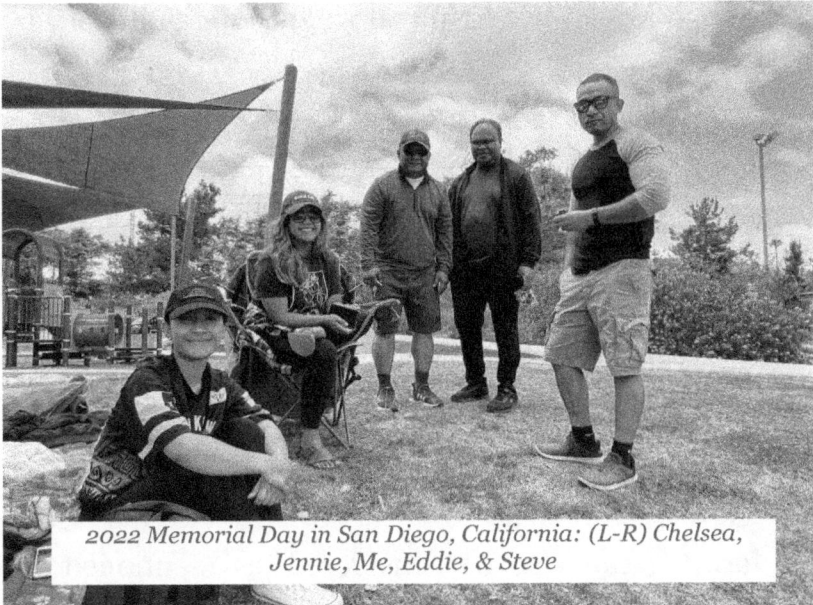

2022 Memorial Day in San Diego, California: (L-R) Chelsea, Jennie, Me, Eddie, & Steve

Following are the steps that we can follow to deal with stress successfully. All these steps are centered on caring for ourselves during a stressful event. They can help us achieve physical, psychological, and emotional well-being during stressful times.

Exercises:

You must have noticed that your head gets heavy when you feel unsettled or face a stressful situation. Because of the hormones, our brain starts releasing while using the glucose triggered by cortisol. When our brain is activated and is constantly in fight-or-flight mode, not only do we get psychologically exhausted but also physically tired.

Exercise can always help restore the energy in your body. When you spend your energy exercising, you start feeling good about yourself. It is the same energy you would have used while thinking about your stressful event, but exercising can help you focus on something that pushes you toward better health. The mode of exercise we choose can differ based on our choices, but they all have one focal point: diverting our focus from stressful thoughts to optimistic ones. You can always start with mild exercises, including morning or evening walks. Joining an exercise group or performing tasks like farming can also be considered, as mentioned in the introduction. Walking or exercising helps us clear our mind of all the stressful thoughts, which may not solve our stressful situation but further complicate it.

Meditation:

Meditation helps you focus on yourself rather than the

situations and stressful conditions in your life. It enables you to focus more on yourself than on something that keeps you engaged in self-destructive or negative thoughts. When you meditate, you start unlocking your awareness of yourself and your surroundings.

People use different meditation methods, including chakras, soft music, meditating outdoors, sitting in different mudras, etc., but they all have one central purpose. That unified purpose is to awaken your self-awareness and potential to recover anything you consider a hurdle in your life.

As mentioned above, meditation comes in different forms and methods; it is up to us what method to meditate with and get accustomed to. One of the methods that people widely opt for is praying. Praying is a form of meditation where you sit in a quiet place and pray to a transcendent authority. Prayers, like meditation, have different forms. Some people resort to listening to peaceful worship or spiritual music. Listening to this genre of music calms a person and distracts their mind from the chaotic events in their lives. This soothing effect is the same that meditation has on a person's mind. Hence, meditation helps stressed people declutter their minds and start practicing self-awareness when combined with spiritual music.

Hence, meditation helps us deal with stressful situations by being less reactive. By doing so, we may only be able to change our situation slowly, but we try to change the factors or elements causing them.

When we are less stressed about reducing stressful events and don't have that adrenaline rush, we push every piece to fall back in. Meditation helps us focus on mending something broken rather than thinking about how that something fell apart in the first place.

Coping Strategies:

When you are under stress, what you should do next is find out your coping strategy. This coping strategy can help you become less conscious of the stressful event, which may further complicate things and situations. Like meditation, coping strategies can help divert focus from stressful events. People have different coping strategies, including cleaning the house, watching a good sitcom, or gardening. These coping strategies always include occupying yourself with something pleasurable amidst your stressful situations. You may find it funny, but some people start watching horror and thriller movies when stressed. When they consume movies from these genres, they focus on how the movie's main protagonist will survive. It helps you forget about your situation for the time being and takes you to the world of that protagonist, who is always seeking a way out from someone or something chasing them in the movie.

Although you feel a certain amount of stress while watching such a movie, that stress is irrelevant to your situation. It removes your mental exhaustion before watching a horror movie and helps you focus on the events unfolding on your TV screen or projector.

Coping strategies may also include mental exercises like keeping a journal about your thoughts and shifting your thoughts to something you are grateful for. Being thankful brings a sense of contentment to you, which helps you significantly when experiencing stressful events. When you start focusing on something you are grateful for, you shift your focus from the things that stress you out or make you sad. Another area you should consider working on while building your coping strategy is ensuring you sleep enough daily. When you are sleep-deprived, your mind wanders to places it shouldn't. Other things that may help you have a clean and healthy diet are focusing on your food intake and regulating the amount of sugar and fatty foods you consume.

Taking good care of your health is a step toward getting you out of your stressful situation. It keeps you from falling into the pits where your stressors tend to push you continuously.

Establishing a Support System:

When you are under stress, it is equally vital for you to work on establishing a support system for yourself. When you have a support system, it helps you manage your stress efficiently. Your support system includes family members, spouses, partners, and friends. Your support system can comprise people you trust and feel safe confiding in. You can talk to them about your feelings and thoughts and what is causing you stress in the first place.

Most of the time, we must realize that it's not suggestions or advice we seek but someone to listen to us. When you feel heard by someone, it brings emotional relaxation and makes you feel like you are not alone in your struggle. There are people out there to help you—people you can count on to find healing.

When you feel like you are under a significant amount of stress and nothing can help you out of it, seeking professional help will be the most appropriate step to take. You can always opt for counseling when you feel like your stressful events have surpassed the point of being heard. Sometimes, a certified counselor may help us find the solution we may not get anywhere else.

A certified counselor can help you develop a modified coping strategy. When you start following this coping strategy, it gradually equips you to manage your stress successfully. You should consider that you can't get the solution in just one day; managing stress is a process. The more you work on it, the more it yields fruit.

Managing Your Time:

You will be less likely to face a stressful situation when managing your time. It would be best to allocate specific time to your work tasks to manage your time efficiently. Keeping a delicate balance and time division between personal and professional lives is always helpful in making someone feel less stressed. Managing your time effectively will prevent you from making you feel like you are missing something in your life.

Working according to a schedule makes tasks less cluttered, and it also reduces the chances of tasks overlapping with each other. When you start prioritizing what you should work on immediately and what you can do later, it can keep you from dealing with task pileups.

Stress Releasing Elements:

Stress doesn't only affect our minds; it also spreads its negative influence on our bodies. Managing stress at an earlier stage saves us from developing other diseases in our bodies that are associated with anxiety and depression. Various activities help a person manage their stress. The following is a list of activities that assist in managing stress and improve a person's overall physical and mental health.

Activities Promoting Flexibility and Balance:

Different exercises come to mind when aiming for a certain level of flexibility and balance in our bodies. On top of the list, there would be three main activities that our mind would think of. They include Tai Chi, yoga, and Pilates. These three activities can benefit the human body by allowing it to improve balance through working on strength. Everyone can perform these activities, as they don't come with any restrictions related to age or gender.

Tai Chi:

Tai Chi was a form of martial arts, but with time, people started practicing it to improve their balance and physical strength. Tai Chi also comes in different types, with different levels and modes of practice. A person can also start practicing the form of Tai Chi to which their body is adapted. These various Tai Chi forms include:

1. Hen Tai Chi
2. Yang Tai Chi

3. Wu Tai Chi

4. Sun Tai Chi

5. Hao Tai Chi

Tai Chi doesn't only help the body but also a person's mind by assisting them in improving their bodily functions and strengthening their bodies simultaneously. When you find which form of Tai Chi suits you as a beginner, you can improve your body's strength and balance level by level. These levels include more complex poses and stretching than the previous one, which a person's body can get habitual to after practicing Tai Chi regularly.

Numerous studies have been conducted on the benefits of Tai Chi on human health, which have resulted in the following findings:

1. It helps an individual reduce the stress levels they are experiencing in their lives.

2. It enhances the strength of the legs' muscles.

3. It helps a person improve their bodily functions and their flexibility.

Tai Chi also has some mild modes of exercise that can be performed by people living with disabilities. Hence, Tai Chi is one of the most helpful physical activities for improving a person's physical and mental health.

Yoga:

Nearly everyone knows what yoga is in this modern world, but little do they know that it isn't a newly practiced form of exercise. Yoga has existed for hundreds of years in India, where it originated. It includes various activities centered on attaining different body postures by stretching and performing different poses.

Like Tai Chi, practicing yoga comes in different forms, which include:

1. Iyengar Yoga
2. Sivananda Yoga
3. Ashtanga Yoga

Although these different types of yoga have some unique differentiation points when compared, they are all focused on posture and breathing. Some yoga exercises can be milder than others, which makes them suitable for a beginner—someone who has never practiced yoga before or has some physical restrictions or disabilities post-accident.

Yoga has numerous health benefits, which include:

1. Promoting the betterment of an individual's physical and mental health.
2. Yoga helps an individual strengthen their balance as the exercises are focused on the muscles' strength in a person's lower body, including hips, ankles, and knees.

3. Lowers a person's blood pressure by allowing them to be in a state of stillness, leaving all their tensions behind.

4. Controls the diseases directly or indirectly related to increased blood pressure, such as cardiac attacks or strokes.

5. Provides relief for body pain, including arthritis.

6. Helps an individual to control their anxiety and manage their stress.

Pilates:

It wouldn't be wrong to consider Pilates the mildest exercise on the list. Pilates is based on the idea of general fitness and health improvement. Different forms of Pilates include classical Pilates, mat Pilates, clinical Pilates, reformer Pilates, and contemporary Pilates. Pilates has various health benefits that include:

1. Helping a person improve their posture.

2. Promotes muscle toning.

3. Increases an individual's mobility and helps them strengthen their balance.[4]

Aerobic Exercises:

Aerobic exercises include exercises that condition an individual's cardiovascular health. The word 'aerobic'

---

[4] (2022), Tai chis, Pilates and Yoga, NHS inform
Retrieved from: https://www.nhsinform.scot/healthy-living/keeping-active/activities/tai-chi-pilates-and-yoga

translates into 'with oxygen.' This connection between the activities and breathing is due to the amount of oxygen the muscles utilize to consume energy while performing these exercises.

These aerobic exercises have a range of benefits for an individual's health, which include:

1. They tend to improve cardiovascular health.
2. Tend to lower the risk of heart disease and maintain blood pressure significantly.
3. Increases the amount of HDL in the body, also known as good cholesterol.
4. Assist in maintaining an individual's blood sugar level.
5. Assists in weight loss.
6. Enhances the lung's functionality.[5]

The three main aerobic exercises that we will be discussing here, along with their impact on human health, are:

Cycling:

Cycling is not just aerobic exercise but is also a fun activity. Individuals can bike to their nearest grocery stores, schools, and colleges for fun, which also introduces them to numerous health benefits that they may not be aware of, such as:

---

[5] (2023), Aerobic exercise, Cleveland Clinic
Retrieved from: https://my.clevelandclinic.org/health/articles/7050-aerobic-exercise

1. An individual who engages in cycling can have fewer chances of suffering from cardiovascular diseases.

2. They will be less likely to experience cancer and depression.

3. Cycling helps individuals stay safe from obesity, diabetes, and arthritis.[6]

Swimming:

Swimming is not just aerobic exercise but a very fun-to-do activity that people of all ages enjoy. This is why you must have seen numerous people having pool picnics or parties. However, swimming is an exercise that is not just limited to being performed in pools, as it can also be done in rivers or the ocean, but with caution.

The following are the health benefits of swimming:

a) It helps burn calories, keeping the body weight in check.

b) Swimming tends to alleviate stress.

c) It helps improve coordination, posture, and balance.

d) It boosts the body's flexibility.

e) Has soothing effects on an individual's mind, as it is considered a therapeutic activity with a low impact

---

[6] (2013), Cycling – health benefits, Better Health Channel
Retrieved from:
https://www.betterhealth.vic.gov.au/health/healthyliving/cycling-health-benefits

that strengthens the body and helps people overcome depression after any traumatic event.[7]

Running:

Running is an aerobic exercise with multiple health benefits for a human's mind and body. When a person invests their time and energy into running, it boosts the blood circulation rate in their body. In addition, it also enhances the individual's respiratory system, as it starts functioning twice as hard as before.

By running, you'll find yourself pushing harder than ever. Every morning or evening, you will try to cover more distance or run for five more minutes than usual. You may not know that you are setting yourself up to cross limitations not just on your body but also on your mind.

You may find yourself questioning how running for extra time uplifts limitations that our minds may have. The answer is that when we prepare ourselves for running for those five additional minutes, we are not just pushing our bodies to cross that distance. We train our mind to overcome what it perceives as a challenge. Our mind then pushes our body to run for an extra five minutes. This helps us see our life's

---

[7] (2013), Swimming – Health Benefits, Better Health Channel
Retrieved from:
https://www.betterhealth.vic.gov.au/health/healthyliving/swimming-health-benefits

stressors, similarly preparing us to face and deal with stressful events with an optimistic and productive attitude.

There are numerous health benefits of running for our bodies, such as:

a) Running helps an individual manage their stress.

b) It helps promote the body's ability to deal with tension and stress, which triggers the release of a chemical hormone called norepinephrine. This chemical is responsible for providing relaxation to a stressed mind.

c) Running in the morning or afternoon can help increase the vitamin D level in an individual's body. Vitamin D is known to curb the symptoms responsible for causing stress in an individual.

d) It helps preserve a person's cognitive ability. Running helps reduce the chances of gradual cognitive decline in individuals. Typically, people can experience cognitive decline after they reach the age of 45. However, regular running helps prevent earlier cognitive decline risks.

e) Regular running helps restore the hippocampus, the part of the brain that stores memories and supports learning.

f) It helps the mind relax and boosts the brain's overall functionality.

g) It helps cure insomnia.

h) It boosts productivity levels in individuals. [8]

Besides these activities, other physical activities help individuals maintain their physical and mental health. These activities are mentioned in the following table. However, their results are like those of the activities mentioned above.

Activities	Sub-Types
Strength training	a. Resistance bands b. Weightlifting c. Bench-pressing
Sports	a. Basketball b. Tennis c. Soccer
Cross training	a. Circuit training b. HIIT workouts
Outdoor Activities	a. Rock climbing b. Hiking

---

[8] (2021), 8 Running Benefits for your Body, Brain, and Well-Being, Cigna Healthcare

Retrieved from: https://www.cigna.com/knowledge-center/mental-health-benefits-of-running#:~:text=Cardiovascular%20exercise%20can%20create%20new,%2C%20higher%20thinking%2C%20and%20learning.

	c. Kayaking

Getting Adequate Sleep:

According to the National Sleep Foundation, the average adult needs seven to nine sleeping hours per night to function well. When you don't sleep adequately, your mind's function will slow down, and you'll also experience fatigue and lethargy.

When an adult doesn't get enough sleep and must go to work, the following day will only add to that adult's stressors. Feeling sluggish, exhausted, and tired can be our body's symptoms—it tells us that the body needs rest. Sleep deprivation, or insomnia, kills our productivity at work and makes us irritated by the people around us. Doing so can seriously affect our social lives as we push people away. What may follow is self-isolation and depression, pushing us toward satisfying ourselves with other harmful means, such as alcohol consumption and drug usage. Many individuals have insomnia or lack sleep despite trying their best to fall asleep. Sometimes, even going to bed early doesn't help because their minds can still be occupied, preventing them from sleeping. Sleep deprivation can also lead to obesity and chronic depression, which is why it is a must for every individual to get an adequate amount of sleep.

Following are some steps that can help an individual fall asleep quickly and stay asleep for a suitable period:

1. Managing our time and dividing it equally between the tasks that must be prioritized can help us save enough time to sleep. Sometimes, we tend to procrastinate and spend hours doing something unnecessary, leaving us no other option but to decrease our sleep time to finish the tasks. By cutting our sleep, we don't realize we can finish the work, leaving us mentally exhausted for the following day. It isn't uncommon for mental exhaustion to lead us toward physical exhaustion as we repeat the same sleepless cycle.

2. Keeping your bed and sheets clean and improving sleep hygiene can help some fall asleep quickly.

3. A fixed schedule for sleeping can help individuals build discipline. It helps them sleep and wake up simultaneously, leading them toward a better timetable for their daily tasks. It tends to increase an individual's productivity level.

4. Opting for a comfortable and cozy mattress and going to bed in comfortable clothing tends to be a great aid in sleeping.

5. Keeping the unnecessary lights off and surrounding oneself in darkness while trying to sleep can make one fall asleep quicker than with lights on.

6. Minimizing our screen time and keeping our phones locked in drawers helps our minds relax before bed.

7. A caffeine-free diet or avoiding caffeine at least three hours before bed can help treat sleeplessness. Consuming nerve-calming tea, such as chamomile tea, has also proven helpful when trying to sleep.

When we have a good sleep cycle, we are less likely to

experience the significant impact of stress. Although everyone feels stressed at some point, the key to dealing with these stresses is often in plain sight. Insomnia or sleeplessness can trigger stressors and often make them look bigger than they are.

Having a Balanced Diet:

When we begin achieving optimal health, we must consider our diet in addition to all the elements above. A diet comprised of fiber, fresh fruits and vegetables, whole grains, foods with unsaturated fats, and omega-3 fatty acids is considered a good diet. A good diet can help us avoid inflammation and bloating, which often damage our tissues, muscles, joints, artery walls, and organs.

We must stop consuming fast and processed food and adopt healthier eating habits. Eating a healthy diet can help our body get a suitable amount of protein, vitamins, and other nutrients instead of filling our bodies with fat when we consume fast food and foods high in sugar.

When we stop eating sugary and processed foods, our bodies gradually stop craving them. This leads us toward a more nutritious diet, such as home-cooked meals, vegetables, and fruits. Eating unhealthily—sugary and fat-induced food— can push us toward high blood sugar levels, increasing our hunger and boosting our blood sugar levels. An increased blood sugar level means increased chances of getting diabetic, which further exposes us to the threats of experiencing cardiovascular issues, dementia, and obesity.

There are other impacts of having a bad diet on our health, such as:

1. Increased chances of suffering from type 2 diabetes

2. Getting exposed to the threat of experiencing breast and colon cancer

3. Depression

4. Having a lower sex drive

5. Increased chances of impotence in males

Benefits of a Healthy Diet:

There are numerous benefits of having a healthy diet:

1. Improves sleeping time and treats insomnia naturally.
2. Improves sex life.
3. Help fight against depression and increase the risk of cardiovascular diseases.
4. Counters the effects of stressful events on our mind and body.
5. Helps sharpen our memories and improve our bodily functions.
6. Improves blood circulation and the digestive system.

7. Boosts our immunity.

8. Helps supply the required nutrients to our brain, heart, bones, muscles, and entire bodily organs.

9. Help fight against osteoporosis and increase chances of suffering from cancer.

10. Helps rejuvenate the skin and adds more years to our life. [9]

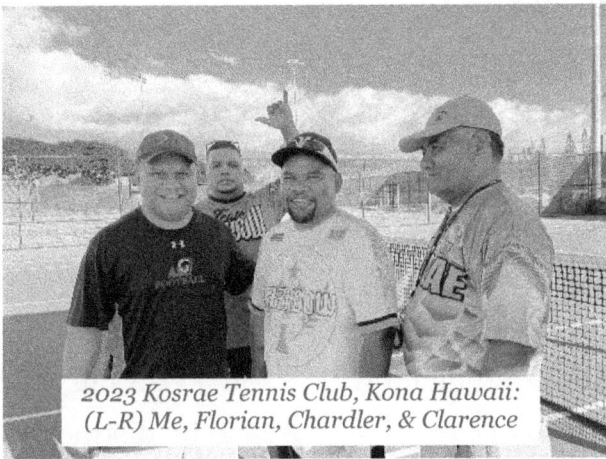

2023 Kosrae Tennis Club, Kona Hawaii: (L-R) Me, Florian, Chardler, & Clarence

Promoting an Active Lifestyle:

When we switch our lifestyles, gear ourselves to lead an active routine, and break the shackles of laziness that we have limited ourselves with, we begin unlocking our true potential and strength—both mental and physical.

Frequent physical activities protect us from developing non-communicable diseases (NCDs). They are called such

---

[9] Staying Healthy, Harvard Health Publishing, Harvard Medical School Retrieved from: https://www.health.harvard.edu/category/staying-healthy

because their initial symptoms aren't as alarming as those of other diseases, but that doesn't decrease their catastrophic impact on our health. NCDs include heart-related health issues like strokes, diabetes, and cancers.

As we mentioned earlier at the beginning of this chapter, cycling, running, swimming, etc., are all means of pushing ourselves toward an active lifestyle.

Benefits of an Active Lifestyle:

The benefits of having an active lifestyle are:

1. It reduces the level of hypertension.
2. Helps in maintaining the body's weight, as mentioned above.
3. Improves our quality of life and boosts our productivity.
4. It helps us keep ourselves sane by distracting us from stressful events.
5. An active lifestyle is also associated with a good mood or the ability to stabilize our mood.[10]

Acquiring Education Regarding Preventative Screening:

When we set ourselves up for a healthy lifestyle, we

---

[10] Physical Activity, World Health Organization
Retrieved from: https://www.who.int/health-topics/physical-activity#tab=tab_1

overlook where we stand on the health scale. We always begin our journey by keeping our future in mind. To achieve our goals for our future, which in this case is attaining optimal health, we must get ourselves checked by physicians and doctors regarding how healthy we are. If we start our journey without knowing what is wrong with our health, we may be setting ourselves up for disheartening experiences and failures.

Example:

You get inspired by an advertisement promoting health on TV or watch your fit neighbor grocery shop at the same supermarket as you do. Now, you are all driven to have a healthy lifestyle and achieve your desired body shape. You start going to the gym, and you start running. You start seeing the results of your consistent workouts and physical activities on your body. Every time you step on a weighing scale, it shows a lower number than the previous one. But suddenly, you experience shortness of breath, which starts mildly but grows stronger as time passes.

After ignoring the issue, you finally decide to visit a doctor. The doctor runs some tests and screenings on you. When you get the results, you will feel disheartened, as your result may show a high sugar level in your blood or weak cardiovascular activity. You may think your efforts to have a fit body have failed. But you wouldn't even believe that it may be the consequence of your previous lifestyle, and although you have a health issue, it may not be as bad as it might have been. Since you haven't done your screening before deciding to switch to a healthy lifestyle, you feel there's nothing more you can do. You make the wrong decision by reverting to your old eating habits and unhealthy lifestyle. Whereas, if you had done your screenings before exercising, running, and eating healthy, you would've been amazed to know that the results in your hands are not as bad as they initially might have been. Therefore, it is always necessary to go for screening and acquire adequate knowledge regarding your current health.

Important Screenings and Tests:

Following is the list of essential screenings and tests that an individual must opt for:

1. Prostate exams/testing.
2. Cholesterol, blood pressure, and blood sugar tests.
3. Skin cancer screenings after consulting a dermatologist.
4. Colorectal cancer screening.
5. Abdominal aortic aneurysm screening.
6. Getting vaccinated for flu, pneumonia, and other diseases.
7. Mental health screenings after consulting a psychiatrist or a psychologist.

8. Vision and hearing exams.

9. Osteoporosis screening for men and women above the age of 65.

10. HIV testing.

11. Physical exams assess overall health and well-being.

12. Seeking consultations from doctors and physicians to discuss risk factors and lifestyle choices.

Physical and Mental Change

Aging is a process that affects not just our skin and bodies but also our minds. As we age, we will notice changes in our appearance and the functionality of our minds and bodies. Depending on how we cater to them, it can range from mild to severe changes. The key is always to take our well-being and health seriously as we age. Aging and the changes it brings to their bodies affect men and women equally. However, this chapter will focus on aging and its effect on men and how their hormonal balance can get disturbed as they get older without considering how a shift is introduced in the male's hormone balance, which triggers the changes in their behavior. Aging is not only associated with the risks of physical health deterioration but also mental health risks.

As humans, we can't stop aging. You may have encountered many people in their late fifties or early sixties who you found more energetic and healthier than those in their early twenties or thirties. We can alter our looks with cosmetic procedures to look younger, but you may keep asking yourself this question: "You look young, but do you feel young?" Until we start feeling young from within, we won't achieve the satisfaction or happiness that we may get from cosmetic procedures done on ourselves. The key always lies in regularly checking your physical and mental fitness.

Following are the changes that an aging male may experience:

Association Between Hormone Imbalance and Physical Changes:

The chemicals in our body are responsible for coordinating different functions in our body. These chemicals are called hormones and carry messages to different body parts through the blood, including your organs, muscles, skin, and tissues. These signals provide indications and instructions to your body. Hormones are of significant value in health maintenance and enhancing the quality of life.

According to various studies by scientists and expert biologists, more than fifty hormones exist in the human body. Hormones are responsible for controlling numerous body functions, which include:

- Metabolism.

- Maintaining an internal balance, i.e., the procedure of homeostasis.
- Keeping sexual health and sexual functionalities in check.
- Influence the sleep cycle.
- Reproduction process.
- Mood stability.
- Growth of the human body and its development.

Hormonal Imbalance:

A person may experience hormonal imbalance when their body produces one hormone excessively while decreasing the production of another hormone. Hormonal disbalance is also associated with numerous health conditions linked to hormones. Increasing and dropping a single hormone can alter many bodily functions. A person experiencing hormonal imbalances may require treatment procedures to regulate the number of hormones in their body. Hormonal imbalances can be temporary or chronic, depending on the severe changes they cause in your body. Some hormonal imbalances may not have a powerful impact on a person's health, but they are known to plummet a person's quality of life.

Health Conditions Triggered by Hormonal Changes:

Hormonal imbalances cause numerous health conditions.

Some of them are mentioned below:

Acne:

A person suffering from hormonal imbalance can experience acne. This acne is called adult acne, as it is not the regular acne that a person experiences during puberty. This adult acne starts appearing on a person's skin when they lack the production of the essential hormones in their body.

Diabetes:

Many individuals have diabetes, which is often triggered by hormonal imbalances. It is one of the significant endocrine conditions in which a person's pancreas produces insufficient insulin. In some cases, although the pancreas produces an adequate amount of insulin, our body may not be able to utilize the amount of insulin being released. There are different types of diabetes, but the most significant are Type 1 diabetes (gestational diabetes) and Type 2 diabetes.

Obesity in Men:

One of the main effects of hormonal imbalance on the physical health of older men is that it causes obesity in them. Numerous hormones send signals to the body when it needs energy from food. They are influential when it comes to utilizing the energy extracted from food, which is why some hormonal imbalances can cause weight gain and fat storage. An increase in cortisol (one of the hormones) and a decrease in hypothyroidism (thyroid hormones) can cause obesity.

Decreased Testosterone (Male Hypogonadism):

Hypogonadism in males is caused by the lack of testosterone produced by the testicles. It has various effects on the male body, including testicular injuries. Lower testosterone also affects the pituitary gland and hypothalamus. When the condition is left untreated for extended periods, it can severely impact male fertility. However, the most suitable treatment available is testosterone replacement therapy. Testosterone is known as the primary androgen, which stimulates characteristic male development and increases the process of spermatogenesis in males. Testosterone helps with:

- Development of sexual organs and genitalia in the male body.
- Moderation of RBCs (Red Blood Cells).
- Strengthening the bones by increasing bone density.
- Providing a boost to reproductive or sexual functions.
- The pituitary gland and hypothalamus control the production or release of testosterone in the testicles.[11]

---

[11] (2022), Low Testosterone (Male Hypogonadism), Cleveland Clinic

Decreased Libido and Fertility Rate:

As mentioned above, a low level of testosterone is linked with a decrease in sperm production, which leads to the risk of male infertility. Alongside the decreased testosterone level, another hormone affects the male fertility rate and reduces sexual desires. Lower estrogen levels in a male body can lower the sexual drive of the person while also plummeting the sperm production rate and decreasing its concentration.

Estrogen is commonly called the *female hormone* despite being present in both males and females. The increase and decrease of this hormone negatively affect a male's body and sexual health. When the level of estrogen increases in a male, it leads to erectile dysfunction. However, when estrogen is lower than the average amount, it causes reduced libido and sexual desires in males. This dysregulation or imbalance in both testosterone and estrogen is naturally associated with aging, but it can be treated with medicines and hormone supplements when necessary. A good diet can also help a person moderate the level of these hormones.[12]

Retrieved from: https://my.clevelandclinic.org/health/diseases/15603-low-testosterone-male-hypogonadism#:~:text=Low%20testosterone%20(male%20hypogonadism)%20is,treatable%20with%20testosterone%20replacement%20therapy.

[12] (2023), The hormones that drive male fertility, Legacy
Retrieved from: https://www.givelegacy.com/resources/the-hormones-that-drive-male-fertility/

Osteoporosis in Men:

Osteoporosis is a bone disease that tends to expand with time. Osteoporosis causes the weakening of bones to the point where they can be easily broken. A person who has osteoporosis can have a higher risk of fractures. According to current studies, testosterone is the hormone responsible for bone health and maintaining its density in males and females. Men with lower testosterone levels are more exposed to the threat of osteoporosis. However, there are still confirmations to be made about the direct link between testosterone and bone health.

When men start aging, they start experiencing a steady decline in hormone levels compared to aging women experiencing menopause. According to the studies, testosterone levels tend to decrease by 1% in men annually after they cross their thirties or forties. The studies have also suggested that bone mineral density in men is closely associated with the level of testosterone. [13]

---

[13] Osteoporosis, Causes, NHS
Retrieved from:
https://www.nhs.uk/conditions/osteoporosis/causes/#:~:text=too%20much%20dieting-,Men,with%20low%20levels%20of%20testosterone.

Testosterone Linked with Other Health Issues in Men:

An imbalance in the testosterone level causes several other health issues in men. These health issues tend to get more severe among aging men. Such health issues include:

A lower energy level and decreased motivation to carry out daily functions.

Testosterone imbalance can lead to men experiencing stress and anxiety, which get more intense as they age.

The lower testosterone level is also said to be linked with obesity, which is one of the significant reasons why older males are exposed to the risk of heart failure, strokes, and diabetes.[14]

Mental Health Risks & Benefits Associated with Aging:

When people start aging, they start facing numerous challenges in their lives, regardless of their gender. These challenges often result from the changes introduced in their lives after they cross their late forties or fifties. These mobility, vision, and functionality changes often affect their mental

---

[14] Daniel Yetman (2022), Is there a link between Testosterone level and osteoporosis, Healthline
Retrieved from: https://www.healthline.com/health/testosterone-and-osteoporosis

health. They find it hard to cope with challenging situations and the loss of people they love. They find it difficult to process the grieving period, which often affects their mental health. One of the significant causes of older men's deteriorating mental health is their loneliness. They find it difficult to relate to the younger generations as they age. They often feel left out by their children, making them irritable toward other people. Such feelings of loneliness and grief often pave the way for these older men to experience depression and anxiety, worsening their mental health.[15]

Besides an increased risk of anxiety and depression, older men also experience a decline in their cognitive functioning. One of the significant causes of older people not being able to recognize people and things and losing their memories is dementia. The cognitive decline in older men can be caused by a variety of reasons, which may include:

Side effects of medicines that older males are on

- Early onset of Alzheimer's disease

- Depression

- Sudden emotional trauma

---

[15] Older Adults and Mental Health, Mental Health Information (National Institute of Mental Health)
Retrieved from: https://www.nimh.nih.gov/health/topics/older-adults-and-mental-health

The cognitive decline in older people can be caused by endocrine disbalance or any side effect of a severe illness or infection, such as COVID-19 contamination or a urinary tract infection. Many adult males start experiencing dementia but are often unaware of it because of its mild initial symptoms.

Evaluating the cognitive ability of older males can help provide numerous health benefits, including therapy or lowering their medicine intake that is triggering cognitive impairment.

According to the studies conducted on the subject, approximately 40% of physicians were unable to detect the symptoms of dementia in their patients. If the symptoms are detected earlier, the necessary measures can be taken to help patients overcome the early symptoms of dementia.

Alzheimer's disease is one of the major threats associated with aging. It causes partial or complete memory loss when it progresses from its initial stages. Unfortunately, there aren't any inventions in the medical world that can reverse the effects of Alzheimer's disease. The only thing that can make an Alzheimer's patient's life easier is the earliest disease detection.

To avoid all the setbacks that older people may face, they should start working toward improving their quality of life.

When an aging person develops a new hobby or interest, it helps them stay happy. By investing their time in creating new hobbies, older people can feel a surge of happiness and fulfillment.

Getting better at their new interest or hobby rewards them with a feeling of accomplishment. Investing time in pursuits can help reduce the level of stress in adults, which is one of the major causes of other diseases.

Older people's mental and physical health can improve with a healthy diet. People should turn toward healthier and more nutritious diets as they age rather than relying on sugary and processed foods. A clean diet helps aging people feel healthier and have an active lifestyle, as an unhealthy diet is associated with an increased risk of obesity. Obesity in older people can easily lead them to face severe cardiovascular health deterioration, including heart strokes and higher chances of heart attacks. Spending time with older people can help them feel important to their children. When people start aging, they feel lonely, which can often transition into depression. Older people have abundant wisdom to share with the younger generation, and they can be better guides for more youthful people when they feel stuck in certain situations brought about by life. Elders can help younger people with the level of wisdom they have by using the experiences they have had in their lives during similar situations, which can be their more significant contribution to society. Appreciating life and older people's relationships can be vital to remaining happy. By being grateful for what they have, they can focus less on what they lack, which brings a feeling of contentment to them.

As mentioned above, developing healthy habits such as mild exercise and a nutritious diet can be significantly helpful. Physical activity can help older people stay fit and speed up their metabolism. Older people can still find meaning in their lives even after spending the years of their childhood and adulthood. What they have is something that a younger generation lacks, and that is their wisdom and their experiences. By sharing their experiences with younger people, older people can help and guide them in a way they can't themselves.

Older people can start being social with others, including their children, neighbors, and people the same age as them. They can have their social group where they can enjoy talking or engaging in activities they like. This social group can provide them with a support system and people they can rely

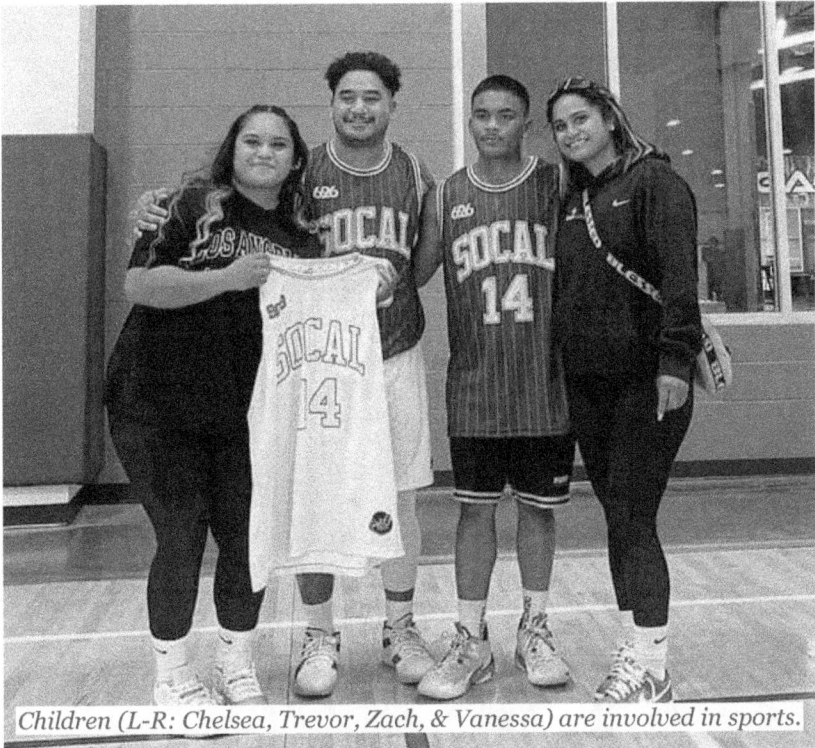

Children (L-R: Chelsea, Trevor, Zach, & Vanessa) are involved in sports.

on in an emergency. Besides that, there will always be people with whom older people can share their feelings. Often, bubbled-up feelings can cause emotional distress. Emotional distress can turn into physical pain if not appropriately addressed. Hence, having a social or support group helps older people get social and provides a means of releasing their emotions. Older people's mental and emotional health tends to be more linked to each other than younger people's mental and emotional health. Other things that can assist older people in having better health are:

- Having regular health screenings and tests to have an early diagnosis of diseases, if any,
- Taking an adequate amount of rest.
- Having sufficient sleep.
- Staying in contact with family and friends.
- Looking for learning opportunities, stop focusing on their age, as many older people can still participate in sports, dance competitions, or martial arts.[16]

[16] Exercise: 7 benefits of regular physical activity, Mayo Clinic
Retrieved from: https://www.mayoclinic.org/healthy-lifestyle/fitness/in-depth/exercise/art-20048389

Key Points Checklist for Chapter 1: Benefits and Challenges

1. **Identify Stress Triggers**: Pay attention to how your body reacts to stress and pinpoint the triggers. Understanding what causes your stress is the first step to managing it effectively.

2. **Regular Exercise**: Incorporate regular exercise into your routine. Physical activity can help manage stress levels and improve physical and mental well-being.

3. **Mindfulness Techniques**: Practice meditation or mindfulness to enhance self-awareness and reduce stress. These practices can provide a sense of calm and balance that benefits your emotional and physical health.

4. **Healthy Coping Strategies**: Develop and implement healthy coping strategies. Engaging in activities you enjoy or maintaining a gratitude journal can significantly help manage stress.

5. **Prioritize Sleep and Balanced Diet**: Prioritize sleep and nutrition. A consistent sleep schedule and a balanced diet are essential for managing stress and promoting overall health.

Call to Action:

Now that we've explored the benefits and challenges, it's time to implement this knowledge. Here's your five-step action plan:

1. **Identify Your Stress Triggers**: Start observing how your body responds to stress and identify the triggers. This awareness is crucial in developing effective stress management strategies.

2. **Embrace Regular Exercise**: Incorporate physical activity into your daily routine. Exercise improves physical health, significantly reduces stress, and enhances mental well-being.

3. **Practice Mindfulness**: Dedicate daily time to practice mindfulness or meditation. These techniques can help manage stress, improve focus, and promote a sense of calm.

4. **Develop Healthy Coping Mechanisms**: Engage in activities that bring you joy or maintain a gratitude journal as part of your stress management strategy. Healthy coping mechanisms can significantly aid in managing stress levels.

5. **Prioritize Your Health**: Sleep well and maintain a balanced diet. These are critical components in managing stress and promoting overall health.

Understanding the benefits and challenges is critical to effectively managing your stress levels. By implementing this checklist, you can take control of your stress and improve your overall well-being. Remember, every step counts on this journey. Let's commit to this action plan and positively impact our health!

Chapter 2: Obesity & Nutrition

"The hardest exercise for most of us fat people is one where we push our chair back from the dinner table."

~ Dolly Pardon

Obesity: Causes, Risks, and Management

Introduction to Obesity

Definition of obesity

Obesity, as defined by the World Health Organization (WHO), is when an individual has an excessive or abnormal accumulation of body fat that may endanger their health.[17] This condition is measured using a metric known as the Body Mass Index (BMI), calculated by dividing a person's weight in kilograms by the square of their height in meters. A BMI of 30 or above is classified as obesity.

The prevalence of obesity has increased to epidemic proportions on a global scale. As of 2016, over 1.9 billion adults aged 18 and over were overweight, with over 650 million being obese. Compared to figures from 1975, we see a near-tripling of worldwide obesity rates. This issue is not

---

[17] Obesity, WHO, Retrieved from: https://www.who.int/health-topics/obesity

restricted to adults alone. In 2020, approximately 39 million children under 5 were overweight or obese, and over 340 million children and adolescents aged between 5-19 were overweight or obese in 2016.[18]

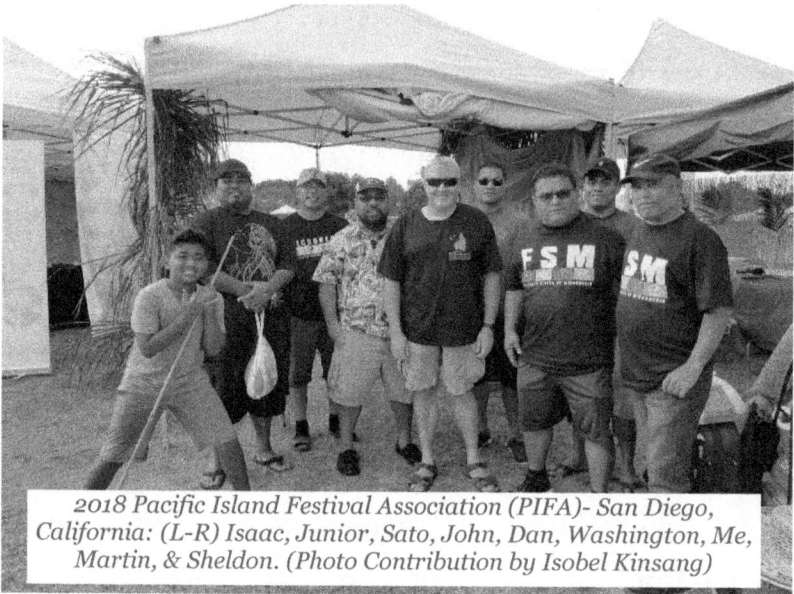

2018 Pacific Island Festival Association (PIFA)- San Diego, California: (L-R) Isaac, Junior, Sato, John, Dan, Washington, Me, Martin, & Sheldon. (Photo Contribution by Isobel Kinsang)

The health implications of obesity are severe and far-reaching. Obesity increases the risk of developing chronic diseases, including cardiovascular diseases like heart disease and stroke, the leading causes of death worldwide. Other health complications include diabetes, musculoskeletal disorders such as osteoarthritis, and certain types of cancer, such as endometrial, breast, ovarian, prostate, liver,

---

[18] Obesity and Overweight, WHO, Retrieved from: https://www.who.int/news-room/fact-sheets/detail/obesity-and-overweight

gallbladder, kidney, and colon cancer.

Several factors contribute to the high prevalence of obesity. Changes in dietary patterns, characterized by increased consumption of energy-dense foods high in fat and sugars, are a significant contributor. Sedentary lifestyles leading to physical inactivity, urbanization, genetic predisposition, cultural aspects, and the availability of unhealthy food choices are other contributing factors.

The impact of obesity varies across different populations and regions. Notably, low- and middle-income countries grapple with a "double burden" of malnutrition, where undernutrition and obesity co-exist within the same communities and households. Urban settings, especially in Africa, have seen a 24% increase in overweight children under five since 2000.

Obesity significantly diminishes the quality of life for individuals and populations. It increases the risk of premature death, disability, and various physical and psychological health issues. Obese individuals may experience breathing difficulties, hypertension, an increased risk of fractures, and early markers of cardiovascular disease. Economically, obesity-related diseases place a considerable burden on healthcare systems worldwide.

Addressing obesity requires a multi-faceted approach that promotes healthy diets, increases physical activity, and creates supportive environments and communities. This involves reducing processed foods' fat, sugar, and salt content, ensuring the availability and affordability of healthy food choices, and implementing policies restricting the marketing of unhealthy foods, particularly to children and teenagers.

Real-life examples underscore the impact of obesity on different populations. The rise in childhood obesity rates in low- and middle-income countries exposes children to the health risks associated with obesity while undernutrition issues persist. Additionally, the global increase in obesity rates reflects the influence of societal and environmental factors on individuals' lifestyle choices and health outcomes.

In summary, obesity is a significant global health issue with far-reaching consequences. Comprehensive strategies and interventions at individual, societal, and policy levels are required to address its prevalence and mitigate its impact on individuals and populations worldwide.

Causes of Obesity
Genetic factors and their role in obesity.
While lifestyle choices contribute to obesity, genetics also play a pivotal role. Recent research suggests that variants in

several genes may contribute to obesity by increasing hunger and food intake. These genetic changes occur too slowly to be solely responsible for the obesity epidemic. However, in some cases, a specific variant of a single gene can cause inherited obesity within a family, underscoring the importance of genetics in understanding this complex disease.

Environmental factors contributing to obesity.

The environment in which we live also plays a significant role in obesity. Unhealthy diets, sedentary lifestyles, and metabolic disorders are critical contributors to the development of obesity. Moreover, social determinants of health (SDOH), such as the availability and affordability of healthy food options, social support, marketing and promotion, and community design, can significantly impact obesity rates.[19] For instance, living in a neighborhood with limited access to fresh produce and safe spaces for physical activity can create an "obesogenic" environment that promotes weight gain.

The interaction between genetics and the environment.

The interaction between genetics and the environment is crucial in understanding obesity. A person with a genetic

---

[19] Causes of Obesity, CDC Retrieved from: https://www.cdc.gov/obesity/basics/causes.html

predisposition to obesity may be more susceptible to weight gain in an obesogenic environment that promotes unhealthy eating habits and a sedentary lifestyle.

Real-life examples offer valuable insights into this complex interaction. Consider a comprehensive study conducted on the island of Kosrae (where I am originally from), one of the four states in the Federated States of Micronesia (FSM); it was found that 88% of adults aged 20 or older are overweight, 59% are obese, and 24% are extremely obese.[20] This astonishing prevalence of obesity has led researchers to explore genetic factors contributing to this health crisis. A census of Kosrae's entire adult population was completed, including individual DNA samples, individual-level data on height, weight, blood pressure, glucose levels, and information about family members' identity and medical status. The goal was to establish the possible relationship between genetic variation and human obesity. The results of these ongoing studies suggest that obesity is a highly heritable trait in this population.

Yet, genetics alone do not account for the rapid increase in obesity rates in the FSM. Environmental factors, such as

---

[20] Cassels S. Overweight in the Pacific: links between foreign dependence, global food trade, and obesity in the Federated States of Micronesia. Global Health. 2006 Jul 11;2:10. doi: 10.1186/1744-8603-2-10. PMID: 16834782; PMCID: PMC1533815.

changes in diet and lifestyle influenced by foreign dependence and global food trade, also play a significant role. Over the past century, the FSM has undergone substantial social change, mainly due to its history of foreign rule and dependence on foreign aid. This has shifted from traditional diets rich in local produce and seafood to more processed foods high in sugar and fat.

Moreover, the Pacific tuna trade exacerbates the obesity epidemic in the FSM. The region's dependence on imported foods, coupled with the ease of global food trade, has resulted in poor dietary choices and increased obesity rates. Despite the abundant fish in the surrounding waters, most locally caught tuna is exported, while the population relies heavily on imported, processed food.

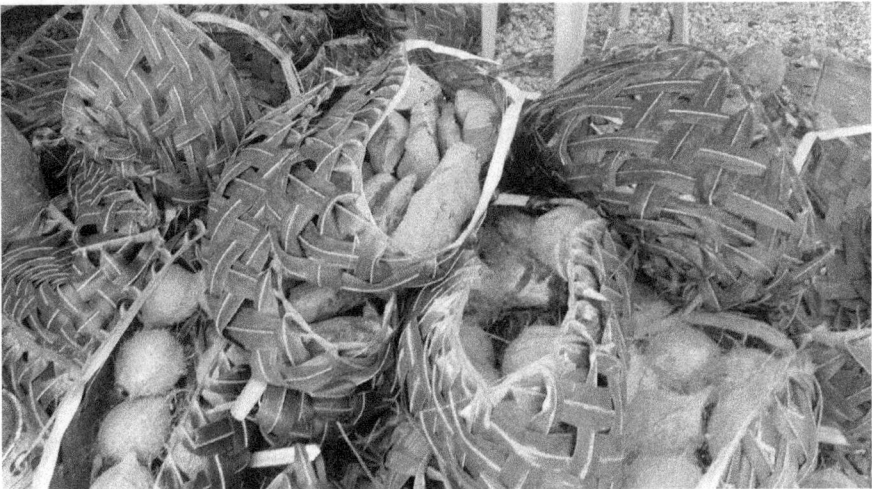

Home grown Crops: cobra, taro, & breadfruit in local baskets

While there is a vital genetic component to obesity in the FSM, environmental factors significantly contribute to the region's high obesity rates. The interplay between genetic predisposition and an obesogenic environment, characterized by unhealthy dietary habits and sedentary lifestyles, underscores the complexity of addressing this health crisis. A multifaceted approach that includes improving the nutritional quality of available foods, promoting physical activity, and addressing the economic and social factors contributing to obesity is required to tackle this issue effectively.

This is one of the many cases where a person (s) with a genetic predisposition to obesity lives in a neighborhood with limited access to healthy food options and opportunities for physical activity. In such a scenario, the interplay between genetic and environmental factors can lead to obesity.

Case studies highlight the causes of obesity.

Addressing the root causes of obesity requires a concerted effort from policymakers, healthcare professionals, and individuals. Policymakers can implement strategies to improve the nutritional quality of food and beverages in public facilities and worksites. They can also create or modify environments to make it easier for people to engage in physical activity.

Healthcare professionals, on the other hand, play a crucial role in educating individuals about healthy eating patterns and the importance of regular physical activity. Lastly, individuals can make conscious choices to adopt healthier lifestyles and seek support from healthcare professionals and community programs.

Understanding the complex interplay between genetics and the environment is critical in tackling obesity. By working together, stakeholders can effectively address this global health crisis, promoting overall health and well-being.

Risks Associated with Obesity

Physical Health Risks of Obesity:
Cardiovascular Diseases

Obesity is a significant risk factor for cardiovascular diseases, the leading cause of death worldwide.[21] The excess weight strains the heart and blood vessels, leading to high blood pressure, elevated cholesterol levels, and an increased risk of heart attacks and strokes.[22]

Type 2 Diabetes

There's a strong link between obesity and type 2 diabetes.

---

[21] World Health Organization. Obesity and overweight. Available from: https://www.who.int/news-room/fact-sheets/detail/obesity-and-overweight (accessed Oct 20, 2023).
[22] Cassels S. Overweight in the Pacific.

Excessive body fat interferes with the body's ability to use insulin correctly, causing insulin resistance and elevated blood sugar levels.[23]

High Blood Pressure
Obesity increases the risk of developing high blood pressure or hypertension. The extra weight necessitates more blood to supply oxygen and nutrients to tissues, increasing pressure on artery walls.[24]

Certain Cancers
Obesity is associated with a heightened risk of several types of cancer, including endometrial, breast, ovarian, prostate, liver, gallbladder, kidney, and colon cancer.[25]

Musculoskeletal Disorders
Excess weight stresses joints, increasing the risk of musculoskeletal disorders like osteoarthritis. Back pain and joint pain are also more common in people with obesity.[26]

Mental Health Risks of Obesity
Obesity can significantly affect mental health, with links to depression, anxiety, and low self-esteem. The social stigma and discrimination associated with weight can further

---

[23] ibid.
[24] ibid.
[25] ibid.
[26] ibid.

contribute to mental health issues.[27]

Other Health Risks

Obesity can lead to sleep apnea, asthma, reproductive complications, and non-alcoholic fatty liver disease (NAFLD). It's also associated with a higher risk of premature death.[28]

Maintaining a Healthy Weight

Maintaining a healthy weight is crucial for overall well-being. Adopting a balanced and nutritious diet, including plenty of fruits, vegetables, whole grains, lean proteins, and healthy fats, is recommended. Regular physical activity is also essential, aiming for at least 150 minutes of moderate-intensity weekly exercise.[29] Additionally, avoiding excessive consumption of sugary and high-fat foods and beverages is vital.

Understanding the immediate and long-term health risks of obesity can help individuals make informed choices to prevent and manage this condition, leading to healthier and more fulfilling lives.

The Link Between Obesity and Other Diseases

The link between obesity and various diseases is an issue of paramount importance in the world of health research today.

---

[27] ibid.
[28] ibid.
[29] ibid.

With obesity rates rising globally, understanding these connections can empower us to address and manage these serious health concerns.

Obesity, defined as an abnormal or excessive accumulation of body fat, is much more than a standalone health condition. It acts as a potent risk factor for severe diseases and health conditions.[30]

Cardiovascular Diseases (CVD) are perhaps one of the most notable health risks associated with obesity. The extra weight accompanying obesity strains the heart and blood vessels, leading to high blood pressure, increased cholesterol levels, and a heightened risk of heart attacks and strokes.[31]

A strong connection also exists between obesity and Type 2 Diabetes. Excess body fat interferes with the body's ability to use insulin correctly, leading to insulin resistance and elevated blood sugar levels.[32] It's noteworthy that alongside rising obesity rates, we have observed a parallel increase in rates of diabetes.[33]

---

[30] Health Effects of Overweight and Obesity, Retrieved from: https://www.cdc.gov/healthyweight/effects/index.html
[31] The Medical Risks of Obesity, PMC, Retrieved from: https://www.ncbi.nlm.nih.gov/pmc/articles/PMC2879283/
[32] Health Risks of Overweight & Obesity, NIDDK, Retrieved from: https://www.niddk.nih.gov/health-information/weight-management/adult-overweight-obesity/health-risks
[33] Obesity, WHO, Retrieved from: https://www.who.int/health-topics/obesity

Furthermore, obesity has been linked to certain types of cancer, including endometrial, breast, ovarian, prostate, liver, gallbladder, kidney, and colon cancers.[34] While the mechanisms behind this connection are still being explored, it's clear that maintaining a healthy weight can significantly reduce the risk of developing these cancers.

Another strong link is seen between obesity and musculoskeletal disorders such as osteoarthritis, where excess weight places additional stress on joints. Back pain and joint pain are also more common in individuals with obesity.[35]

In addition, obesity can lead to conditions like sleep apnea, asthma, and non-alcoholic fatty liver disease (NAFLD).[36] In children, obesity increases the risk of contributing to cardiovascular disease, such as high cholesterol and high blood pressure.[37]

These connections underscore the importance of addressing obesity through comprehensive health and lifestyle interventions to reduce the burden of these associated

[34] Health Risks Linked to Obesity, WebMD, Retrieved from: https://www.webmd.com/obesity/obesity-health-risks
[35] Fast Facts – Obesity-Related Chronic Disease, GWU, Retrieved from: https://stop.publichealth.gwu.edu/fast-facts/obesity-related-chronic-disease
[36] Obesity Medicine - Which Diseases Are Related to Obesity?, Retrieved from: https://obesitymedicine.org/diseases-related-to-obesity/
[37] Obesity and Chronic Diseases, UMC, Retrieved from: https://www.umc.edu/Research/Centers-and-Institutes/Centers/Mississippi-Center-for-Obesity-Research/Resources/Obesity_and_Chronic_Diseases.html

diseases. Our collective mission is to combat this global health concern, emphasizing the positive impact of maintaining a healthy weight on overall well-being.

Mental Health Implications of Obesity

In our ongoing exploration of obesity and its health implications, we've examined numerous physical conditions linked to this health concern. However, the conversation would be incomplete without addressing an equally important aspect - the mental health implications of obesity.

Obesity, characterized by an abnormal or excessive accumulation of body fat, is not just a physical health issue. It can profoundly affect an individual's psychological well-being, shaping their emotional health and overall quality of life.[38]

Research indicates that individuals with obesity are at an increased risk of various mental health disorders, including depression, anxiety, and eating disorders.[39] These conditions can create a vicious cycle, as the emotional distress might lead to behaviors like overeating, contributing to further weight

---

[38] Causes and Consequences of Obesity, WHO, Retrieved from: https://www.who.int/news-room/questions-and-answers/item/obesity-health-consequences-of-being-overweight

[39] Link Obesity and Mental Health, Retrieved from: https://www.ncbi.nlm.nih.gov/pmc/articles/PMC6052856/

gain.[40]

Depression, one of the most common mental health disorders globally, is significantly more prevalent among individuals with obesity. This association is thought to be influenced by a complex interplay of biological, psychological, and social factors.[41]

Anxiety disorders, too, show a strong link with obesity. The social stigma and discrimination associated with obesity can lead to heightened worry, unease, and fear, manifesting in various forms of anxiety.[42]

Eating disorders, such as binge eating disorder, bulimia nervosa, and night eating syndrome, are also more common in individuals with obesity. These conditions involve repeated episodes of excessive food consumption, often in response to stress or negative emotions.[43]

Moreover, obesity can impact self-esteem and body image, leading to feelings of shame, guilt, and low self-worth. This

---

[40] Eating Disorder, National Institute of Mental Health, Retrieved from: https://www.nimh.nih.gov/health/topics/eating-disorders/index.shtml

[41] Why People Become Overweight, Harvard Medical School, Retrieved from: https://www.health.harvard.edu/staying-healthy/why-people-become-overweight

[42] Depression and Anxiety, WebMD, Retrieved from: https://www.webmd.com/depression/depression-or-anxiety

[43] Binge-eating Disorder, Mayo Clinic, Retrieved from: https://www.mayoclinic.org/diseases-conditions/binge-eating-disorder/symptoms-causes/syc-20353627

negative self-perception can impair social relationships, occupational functioning, and overall life satisfaction.[44]

Understanding the mental health implications of obesity is crucial for holistic care. It highlights the need for integrated treatment approaches that address both the physical and mental health aspects of obesity.

Promoting mental well-being is integral to our mission of combating obesity. By acknowledging and addressing these mental health implications, we can empower individuals to break free from the cycle of obesity and lead healthier, happier lives.

Statistical Data on Obesity-Related Health Risks

Obesity is not merely a health issue individuals face but a global epidemic that carries significant societal and individual burdens. It's an invisible chain that binds millions worldwide, impacting lives across all age groups and geographies. The narrative of obesity is etched in statistics, but behind these numbers are real people, real struggles, and real implications.

According to the World Health Organization, in 2017 alone, over 4 million lives were lost due to consequences directly

---

[44] Emotional Toll, Retrieved from:
https://www.healthychildren.org/English/health-issues/conditions/obesity/Pages/The-Emotional-Toll-of-Obesity.aspx

associated with being overweight or obese.[45] This sobering statistic underscores the urgent need for action.

The prevalence of obesity has seen a dramatic rise over the decades. In 2016, more than 1.9 billion adults aged 18 years and older were overweight, of which over 650 million were obese. Nearly 40% of adults carried more weight than their body frames were designed to bear. This paints a stark picture of the scale of the challenge we face.

Children are not immune to this health crisis either. In 2020, 39 million children under 5 were overweight or obese. Furthermore, the prevalence of overweight and obesity among children and adolescents aged 5-19 has surged from just 4% in 1975 to more than 18% in 2016.

Let's, again, take a closer look at the Federated States of Micronesia (FSM), where the obesity rates are particularly alarming. In Kosrae, one of the four states in the FSM, a staggering 88% of adults aged 20 or older are overweight, 59% are obese, and 24% are extremely obese.[46] This small island nation encapsulates the global struggle against obesity, highlighting this epidemic's multifaceted causes and impacts.

Obesity is a significant risk factor for many chronic

---

[45] Obesity and Overweight, WHO, Retrieved from: https://www.who.int/news-room/fact-sheets/detail/obesity-and-overweight
[46] Cassels S. Overweight in the Pacific.

diseases, including cardiovascular diseases, diabetes, and certain types of cancer.[47] It's also associated with musculoskeletal disorders, such as osteoarthritis. The risks increase even when a person is only slightly overweight.

The causes of obesity are multifactorial. At its core, it results from an imbalance between calories consumed and expended.[48] Changes in global diets, increased consumption of energy-dense foods high in fat and sugars, and decreased physical activity have fueled the rise in obesity rates.[49]

Despite efforts to address this epidemic, no country has yet succeeded in reversing its growth, according to the WHO.[50] This narrative underscores the need for comprehensive strategies to prevent and manage obesity. It calls for a global, regional, and national commitment to tackle this public health challenge head-on.

Health Impacts of Obesity
The impact of obesity on cardiovascular health.

We are shedding light on an overlooked integral aspect of health - the link between obesity and cardiovascular health. It's a topic that affects millions worldwide. "The CDC 2022

---

[47] Obesity and Overweight, WHO
[48] ibid.
[49] ibid.
[50] ibid.

Adult Obesity Prevalence Maps for 50 states, the District of Columbia, and 3 US territories show the proportion of adults with a body mass index (BMI) equal to or greater than 30 (≥30 kg/m2) based on self-reported weight and height."[51] [See Fig. 2-1] Our mission today is to help you understand its implications.

Map: Overall Obesity

Prevalence[†] of Obesity Based on Self-Reported Weight and Height Among U.S. Adults by State and Territory, BRFSS, 2022

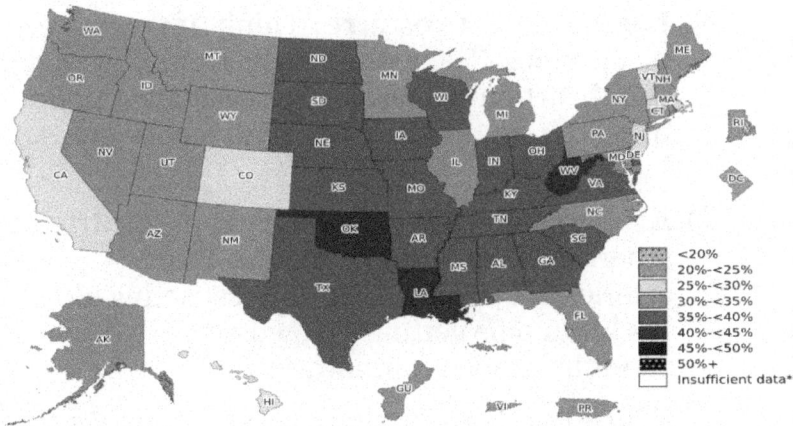

[Fig. 2-1]

Obesity, characterized by excessive body fat, does more than weigh you down physically. It carries significant heart and blood vessel risks, catalyzing various cardiovascular

---

[51] Adult Obesity Prevalence Maps, CDC, Retrieved from https://www.cdc.gov/obesity/data/prevalence–maps.html

diseases. Here are some key examples to help illustrate this:

a) **Heart Disease**: Picture your heart as the engine that powers your body. When carrying extra weight, your heart must work harder, like an engine pulling a heavier load. This strain can lead to conditions like heart failure and heart attacks.

b) **Stroke**: Imagine a busy highway suddenly blocked by an accident. That's akin to what happens during a stroke. Obesity increases the risk of blood clot formation, which can block the blood supply to your brain, causing a stroke.

c) **High Blood Pressure**: Think of your arteries as blood pipes. The extra weight from obesity makes your heart pump harder, increasing the pressure in these pipes, leading to high blood pressure or hypertension.

d) **Atherosclerosis**: Obesity can contribute to atherosclerosis, where plaque builds up in your arteries, narrowing them and restricting blood flow. It's like a pipe getting clogged over time, which can result in various complications.

e) **Diabetes**: Obesity significantly increases the risk of type 2 diabetes, boosting the risk of heart disease and stroke. It's a domino effect that starts with excess body weight.

These are just some examples of how obesity impacts cardiovascular health. The purpose is not to alarm you but to inform and empower you. Maintaining a healthy weight through a balanced diet, regular physical activity, and positive lifestyle modifications can significantly reduce these risks.

The role of obesity in diabetes development

Allow me to take you on a journey to a beautiful yet health-challenged part of our world - the Pacific region, specifically the Federated States of Micronesia (FSM). We'll explore the role of obesity in diabetes development, using real-life examples from this area.

Obesity is more than just a matter of carrying extra weight. It's a key player in developing various health conditions, including a global health crisis significantly impacting the Pacific region and FSM: diabetes.

In the Pacific region, the rates of overweight and obesity are alarmingly high. For instance, in Kosrae, a district in FSM, 88% of adults aged 20 or older are overweight, and 59% are obese.[52] Not to throw only my people under the bus, so to speak, but to address a significant problem in the Pacific region.[53] I must also add that it is not just a Pacific region issue but a global issue. This situation has led to an increased risk of developing diabetes at a young age, especially among children and adolescents.

But why does obesity play such a significant role in diabetes development? Obesity is closely associated with insulin

---

[52] Obesity in the FSM, NIH, Retrieved from:
https://pubmed.ncbi.nlm.nih.gov/16834782/
[53] Diabetes Associations in the Pacific, NIH, Retrieved from:
https://www.ncbi.nlm.nih.gov/pmc/articles/PMC7953240/

resistance, a condition where your body doesn't respond well to the insulin it produces. Insulin is like a key that opens the doors of your cells to let sugar (glucose) in. When insulin-resistant, the doors don't open properly, leaving too much sugar in your bloodstream. Over time, this can lead to type 2 diabetes.

One major factor contributing to the obesity epidemic in the Pacific region and the FSM is changing dietary patterns. There's been an increased intake of energy-dense foods high in fat and sugars and decreased physical activity. Imagine exchanging fresh fish and fruits for processed food high in salt, sugar, and unhealthy fats. This significant shift in lifestyle has contributed to the skyrocketing rates of obesity and, consequently, diabetes.

It's worth mentioning that the economic burden of diabetes care is enormous. For instance, in Nauru and the Solomon Islands, diabetes care consumes 20% of annual government healthcare expenditure.[54] These estimates were much higher than the global average.

However, it's not all gloomy. Efforts are underway to address this issue. We can make a difference by promoting healthy eating habits, increasing physical activity, and

---

[54] ibid.

implementing policies to limit the marketing and availability of unhealthy foods.

Remember, every step towards healthier choices is a step away from obesity and diabetes. It's our collective responsibility to ensure a healthier future for the Pacific region, the FSM, and, indeed, the world. Together, we can turn the tide on obesity and diabetes.

Obesity and its effects on mental health

In this section, we're exploring a critical topic that affects millions worldwide and is particularly prominent in the Federated States of Micronesia (FSM) - obesity and its impact on mental health.

Obesity, characterized by excessive body fat, is more than just a physical health issue. It's a condition that can also significantly affect an individual's mental health, leading to depression, anxiety, and low self-esteem.

In the FSM, this issue comes into sharp focus. With 88% of adults being overweight, obesity is alarmingly high.[55] This situation has likely contributed to many mental health challenges within the population.

Despite receiving billions of dollars in foreign aid, sufficient

---

[55] Overweight in the Pacific, NCBI, Retrieved from:
https://www.ncbi.nlm.nih.gov/pmc/articles/PMC1533815

resources have not been directed toward addressing this pressing health issue.[56] One might ask why these funds are not being used more effectively to combat obesity and promote better mental health among the population. This leads us to a broader question: Is this a challenge unique to FSM, or is it reflective of a global issue?

The truth is the situation in the FSM is not an isolated case. Around the globe, many governments struggle with prioritizing and allocating resources to combat obesity and its associated mental health challenges effectively. Despite the clear links between obesity, poor mental health, and overall well-being, these aspects of health often do not receive the attention they deserve.

For instance, let's consider a hypothetical case of a young adult living in a low-income neighborhood in a developed country. They may have limited access to affordable healthy food options or safe spaces for physical activity, increasing their risk for obesity. As their weight increases, they might face social stigma or bullying, leading to mental health issues like depression and anxiety. This example underscores how systemic issues can contribute to the cycle of obesity and poor mental health.

---

[56] ibid.

Addressing the mental health impacts of obesity requires a comprehensive, global approach. This includes education and access to mental health services and implementing policies that promote healthy lifestyles and equitable access to resources.

The FSM serves as a stark reminder of the urgent need for action. Governments and international organizations must recognize obesity as a global public health priority. By doing so, we can allocate resources more effectively, implement strategies that address the root causes, and ultimately improve individuals' physical and mental health outcomes worldwide.

Charts and figures illustrating the health impacts of obesity.

a) The table below shows overweight and comparison data between men and women in the U.S. population:

Prevalence of Overweight and Obesity

Adults

Age-adjusted ⬚ percentage of US adults with overweight, obesity, and severe obesity by sex, 2017–2018 NHANES Data[2]

	All (Men and Women)	Men	Women
Overweight	30.7	34.1	27.5
Obesity (including severe obesity)	42.4	43.0	41.9
Severe obesity	9.2	6.9	11.5

[Fig. 2.2] 2017-2018 NHANES Data[57]

- Nearly 1 in every 3 men (30.7%) is overweight.
- The percentage of overweight men is higher than women.

b) The table below shows a comparison between the general U.S. population and Native Hawaiians and Pacific Islanders general health status:

General Health Status

Figure 2. Age-sex-adjusted percentage of persons of all ages who had excellent or very good health, by Native Hawaiian and Pacific Islander detailed race: United States, 2014

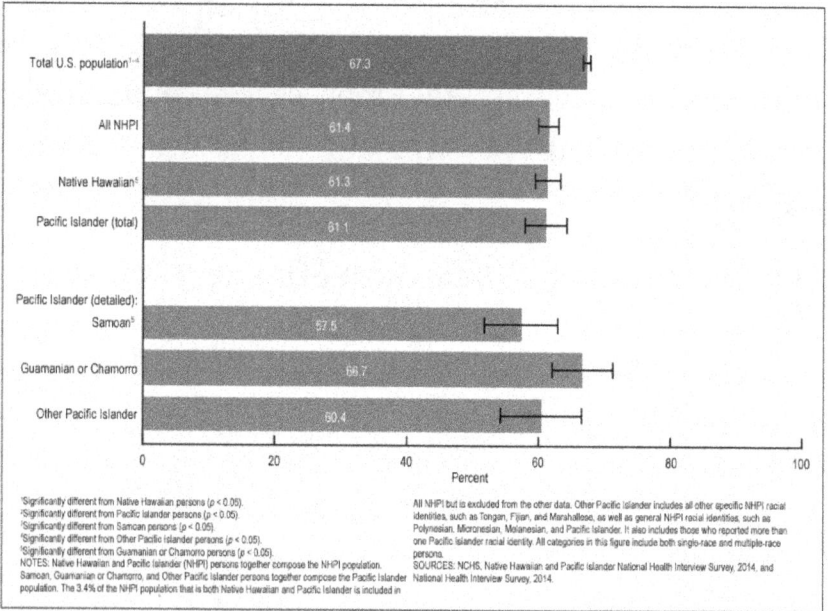

[Fig. 2.3] U.S. Population and NHPI General Health Status.[58]

---

[57] Obesity Charts, Retrieved from: https://www.niddk.nih.gov/health-information/health-statistics/overweight-obesity

[58] Obesity and NHPI, Retrieved from: https://minorityhealth.hhs.gov/obesity-and-native-hawaiianspacific-islanders

If you are interested in further details of the above chart, use this download link for the actual report: https://www.cdc.gov/nchs/nhis/shs/tables.htm

    c) The third and final table for the section on obesity is from a study done by Susan Cassels, which shows a significant increase between 1998 and 2000. [See Fig. 2.4]

Patterns of overweight and obesity in 1988 & 2000

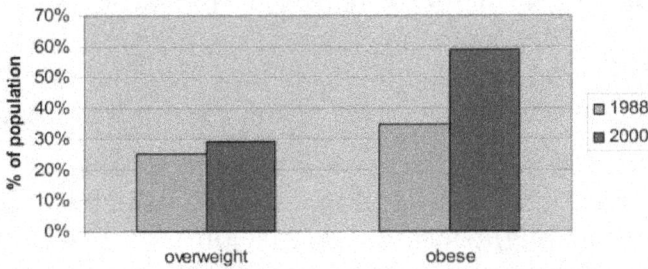

[Fig. 2.4] Overweight in the Pacific.[59]

Managing Obesity
Medical interventions to treat obesity.

The escalating rates of obesity worldwide, including in places like the Federated States of Micronesia (FSM), where 88% of adults are overweight, have made obesity a global health priority. It's about physical health, mental well-being,

---

[59] Susan Cassels, Overweight in the Pacific.

and quality of life.

Thankfully, we're not powerless against this challenge. Effective medical interventions and procedures can help manage and treat obesity. These solutions vary, but all aim to improve an individual's health and well-being.

a) **Healthy Lifestyle Changes**: The first line of defense against obesity usually involves modifying one's lifestyle. This includes eating a balanced, calorie-controlled diet, engaging in regular physical activity, and ensuring adequate sleep. It's like setting the foundation of a house - everything else builds upon it.

b) **Behavioral Weight-Loss Programs**: Sometimes, individuals need a little more support, which is where behavioral weight-loss programs come in. Healthcare professionals work with individuals to develop a personalized plan that combines diet, exercise, and behavioral strategies. It's like having a personal coach guiding you towards your health goals.

c) **Medicines**: When lifestyle changes aren't enough, certain FDA-approved medications can aid in weight loss or management. These medicines work in different ways - some make you feel less hungry, and others make it harder for your body to absorb fat. They're like extra tools to help you on your weight loss journey.[60]

d) **Weight-Loss Devices**: Gastric balloons or bands can sometimes promote weight loss. These medical devices work by limiting how much you can eat or slowing down digestion. Imagine these as physical barriers helping you control your food intake.

---

[60] Behavioral Weight-loss Programs, NHLBI, Retrieved from: https://www.nhlbi.nih.gov/health/overweight-and-obesity/treatment

e) **Weight-Loss Surgery**: Weight-loss surgery might be an option for individuals with a BMI of 35 or greater who face obesity-related complications. Various types of surgeries exist, each with its own benefits and risks. This is akin to a significant renovation project, altering the structure of your digestive system to aid in weight loss.

Remember, while these medical interventions can be effective, they're most successful when combined with ongoing lifestyle changes. It's not just about treating obesity; it's about embracing a healthier way of living.

Lifestyle modifications to prevent and control obesity.

Today, we embark on an essential journey towards understanding lifestyle modifications that can help us manage and overcome obesity. It's a transformation journey, not just for individuals but for entire communities and nations.

The first step on this path is balance. A balanced diet, rich in various nutritious foods, forms the crucial foundation for weight management. Your plate should contain colorful vegetables, fruits, lean meats, protein-rich legumes, and whole grains. At the same time, it's imperative to limit high-calorie, nutrient-poor foods such as processed snacks, refined carbohydrates, and fatty cuts of meat.[61]

---

[61] Lifestyle Modifications for Obesity, NYU Langone Health, Retrieved from: https://nyulangone.org/conditions/obesity/treatments/lifestyle-modifications-for-obesity

Imagine you're at a community event with an assortment of food options. The first option should be for the fresh fruit platter over a bowl of chips or a plate of cookies. This choice isn't just about consuming fewer calories; it's about nourishing your body with essential vitamins and minerals.

Hydration also plays a crucial role in a balanced lifestyle. Water should be your drink, while high-calorie, sugar-laden beverages are best avoided. The next time you feel thirsty, reach for a glass of water instead of a soda.

Yet, a balanced diet is only half the solution. Regular physical activity completes the picture. Whether walking, swimming, or yoga, incorporating moderate activity into your routine can significantly contribute to weight loss and overall health.

Here's a practical tip: Make physical activity a part of your daily life. Choose walking over driving, take the stairs instead of the elevator, and remember to take breaks to walk or stretch during your workday. These small changes can become habits, leading to significant strides in your weight loss journey.

Recognizing that obesity can pose physical limitations, professional guidance can make a difference. Qualified physical therapists can help address physical limitations or health concerns related to exercise, ensuring a safe and effective workout regimen.

More importantly, the fight against obesity calls for concerted action by government leaders. The appropriate allocation of funds towards health promotion initiatives, support for physical education programs in schools, and the creation of safe, accessible spaces for physical activity are just some ways leaders can foster healthier communities.

In conclusion, achieving and maintaining a healthy weight through diet and exercise can help manage obesity and reverse associated conditions like hypertension and type 2 diabetes. Remember, every step you take towards healthier choices is a step away from obesity and towards a healthier nation. We're on this journey together. Let's take these steps one at a time.

It's also important to note that different individuals might require different approaches. For some, lifestyle changes alone may lead to sufficient weight loss. For others, medication or bariatric surgery might be necessary. Always seek professional medical advice to understand the best approach for you.

Let's stand together in this fight against obesity. We have the knowledge, the strategies, and the determination. We can create a healthier future with the proper focus and commitment.

Case studies on successful obesity management.

The global health landscape is witnessing a rising tide of obesity, a chronic condition affecting millions worldwide. As we navigate this challenge, there's no one-size-fits-all solution. Instead, it's through understanding and learning from successful case studies that we can glean effective strategies for managing obesity.

Case Study 1: Obesity in the Federated States of Micronesia (FSM)

The Federated States of Micronesia (FSM), particularly the island of Kosrae, has been grappling with alarming rates of obesity. With 88% of adults aged 20 or older being overweight and 59% being obese, the situation was dire.[62] However, the FSM has turned this crisis into an opportunity to learn and initiate change.

Their approach combined community involvement, policy changes, and lifestyle modifications. The cornerstone involved promoting a balanced diet rich in locally sourced fruits, vegetables, lean meats, and whole grains while limiting high-calorie, nutrient-poor foods. They also emphasized the importance of hydration, encouraging water consumption

---

[62] Susan Cassels, Overweight in the Pacific.

over sugar-laden beverages.[63]

Physical activity was integrated into daily life, with initiatives promoting walking, swimming, and other forms of moderate exercise. These efforts were supplemented by professional guidance from physical therapists to ensure safe and effective exercise regimens for individuals with physical limitations due to obesity.[64]

Governmental intervention also played a crucial role. Funds were allocated towards health promotion initiatives, support for physical education programs in schools, and creating safe, accessible spaces for physical activity. This multi-pronged approach fostered a healthier community and played a significant role in managing obesity.[65]

Case Study 2: Post-Bariatric Surgery Medical Management

Bariatric surgery provides an effective long-term therapy for severe obesity. However, the journey doesn't end there. Post-bariatric care is crucial for maintaining weight loss and overall health.[66]

A comprehensive post-bariatric care program emphasizes

---

[63] ibid.
[64] ibid.
[65] ibid.
[66] Busetto et al. (2017) Practical Recommendations of the Obesity Management Task Force of the European Association for the Study of Obesity for the Post-Bariatric Surgery Medical Management

regular dietary counseling, protein intake and supplementation, and micronutrient supplementation to prevent deficiencies. It also provides guidelines for managing nutritional problems such as food intolerance, vomiting, regurgitation, diarrhea, and steatorrhea.[67]

Monitoring and managing co-morbidities, such as type 2 diabetes, obstructive sleep apnea, dyslipidemia, and hypertension, are crucial before and after bariatric surgery. A multidisciplinary follow-up and the role of primary care in the long-term management of bariatric patients cannot be overstated.[68]

These case studies underscore the importance of a comprehensive, individualized approach to obesity management. They highlight that managing obesity isn't just an individual responsibility but requires concerted efforts from healthcare professionals, government leaders, and communities.

As we continue our journey toward healthier communities and nations, remember that every step toward healthier choices is a step away from obesity. We can transform healthy outcomes and create a healthier future with continued

---

[67] ibid.
[68] ibid.

learning, dedication, and collaboration.

Obesity Summary

We began by defining obesity and examining its prevalence, emphasizing the importance of understanding this issue. We then explored the multifaceted causes of obesity, delving into the interplay between genetic and environmental factors. Through various case studies, we gained insights into real-world scenarios that highlight the causes of obesity.

We also examined the risks associated with obesity. It became evident that the impact of obesity extends beyond physical health, affecting mental well-being, too. From immediate health risks to long-term complications, we discussed the profound link between obesity and other diseases.

We took a closer look at the health impacts of obesity, focusing on cardiovascular health, diabetes, and mental health. The charts and figures we reviewed vividly depicted the significant toll obesity can take on an individual's health.

The subsequent discussion on obesity-related conditions further highlighted the gravity of the situation. We delved into the intricate relationship between obesity and diabetes, cardiovascular disease, and mental health disorders, reinforcing the urgent need for effective management strategies.

In our exploration of managing obesity, we discovered a range of interventions available. From medical treatments and surgical procedures to lifestyle modifications, the case studies we reviewed offered hope and demonstrated that successful obesity management is possible.

As we continue with the book, it's essential to recognize the importance of addressing obesity. The knowledge we've gained about obesity's causes, risks, and management strategies is a powerful tool. Now more than ever, we must encourage further study and proactive measures against obesity.

This is not just about individual health; it's about the health of our communities, nations, and world. Together, we can make a difference. Let's continue to learn, to research, and to act. Let's empower ourselves and others to manage and overcome obesity. The journey may be challenging, but the rewards - healthier, happier lives - are undoubtedly worth it.

.

Nutrition: Healthy Aging from The Inside Out

Eating for Nutrition & Enjoyment:

Aging gracefully starts from the inside out. As men cross the 50-year mark, paying attention to their diet and lifestyle choices becomes increasingly essential. Eating a balanced diet rich in nutrient-dense foods and limiting processed and high-sugar foods can contribute to a healthier and more enjoyable life in later years.

Eat A Variety of Nutrient-Dense Foods

For men over 50, maintaining good health and preventing age-related diseases requires consuming a diverse range of nutrient-dense foods. Nutrient-dense foods are defined as those that offer a significant quantity of essential nutrients, such as vitamins and minerals, relative to the number of calories they contain. Including various fruits, vegetables, whole grains, lean proteins, and healthy fats in the diet can help ensure that the body receives all the necessary nutrients for optimal health.[69] For example, incorporating healthy fruits and vegetables like berries, leafy greens, and tomatoes can provide antioxidants that combat oxidative stress and

---

[69] Harvard T.H. Chan School of Public Health. (n.d.). The Nutrition Source. https://www.hsph.harvard.edu/nutritionsource/healthy-eating-plate/

reduce the risk of chronic diseases.[70] Consuming adequate amounts of lean proteins, such as fish, poultry, beans, and low-fat dairy, can help maintain muscle mass and support overall health.

Limit Processed and High-Sugar Foods

As men age, their metabolism tends to decelerate, making it more challenging to maintain a healthy weight.[71] Overindulging in processed and high-sugar foods can result in weight gain, inflammation, and a higher likelihood of developing chronic health problems such as type 2 diabetes and heart disease.

To support your general well-being and sustain a healthy weight, it's crucial to restrict your consumption of processed and high-sugar foods. This means steering clear of sugary drinks, snacks, and refined carbohydrates that can trigger sudden spikes in blood sugar levels. Instead, go for whole, minimally processed foods that offer consistent energy and help promote healthy aging. In conclusion, adopting a balanced diet rich in nutrient-dense foods and limiting processed and high-sugar foods can significantly contribute to

---

[70] Slavin, J. L., & Lloyd, B. (2012). Health Benefits of Fruits and Vegetables. Advances in Nutrition, 3(4), 506–516. https://doi.org/10.3945/an.112.002154
[71] Mayo Clinic. (2020, February 8). Men's Health: Tips for aging well. https://www.mayoclinic.org/healthy-lifestyle/mens-health/in-depth/mens-health/art-20047764

healthy aging for men over 50. Men can support their overall health and well-being as they age by making mindful choices and enjoying a wide range of nutritious foods.

Include sources of protein, whole grains, fruits, and vegetables in meals

As men enter their fifties and beyond, it becomes progressively more critical to be mindful of the specific components of their diet. Incorporating protein sources, whole grains, fruits, and vegetables into meals can help ensure they receive the necessary nutrients to support optimal health and well-being. Incorporating these food groups into one's diet can aid in maintaining muscle mass, managing a healthy weight, and minimizing the risk of chronic illnesses.

Protein is a critical macronutrient for maintaining and repairing body tissues, including muscles, which tend to decline as men age.[72] Adequate protein intake is essential for preserving muscle mass, contributing to mobility, strength, and overall quality of life. High-quality protein sources for men over 50 include lean meats such as poultry and fish and plant-based options like beans, lentils, and tofu. Incorporating various protein sources into meals can help

---

[72] Wu, G. (2016). Dietary protein intake and human health. Food & Function, 7(3), 1251-1265. https://doi.org/10.1039/C5FO01530H

ensure that men receive all the essential amino acids required for proper bodily function.

Whole grains, such as brown rice, quinoa, oatmeal, and whole wheat bread, are excellent sources of essential dietary fiber, vitamins, and minerals. Including whole grains in your diet has been associated with a decreased likelihood of developing heart disease, type 2 diabetes, and certain types of cancer.[73] The fiber content in whole grains also supports healthy digestion and can help maintain a feeling of fullness, which is beneficial for weight management. Replacing refined grains with whole grains in meals can significantly improve the nutritional quality of the diet.

Including a wide variety of fruits and vegetables in your diet is essential, as they are packed with vital vitamins, minerals, and phytonutrients that can aid in safeguarding against chronic illnesses, boosting the immune system, and improving overall health.[74] Consuming a diverse range of colorful fruits and vegetables can offer essential nutrients like

---

[73] Aune, D., Keum, N., Giovannucci, E., Fadnes, L. T., Boffetta, P., Greenwood, D. C., ... & Norat, T. (2016). Whole grain consumption and risk of cardiovascular disease, cancer, and all cause and cause specific mortality: Systematic review and dose-response meta-analysis of prospective studies. BMJ, 353, i2716. https://doi.org/10.1136/bmj.i2716

[74] Aune, D., Giovannucci, E., Boffetta, P., Fadnes, L. T., Keum, N., Norat, T., ... & Tonstad, S. (2017). Fruit and vegetable intake and the risk of cardiovascular disease, total cancer and all-cause mortality—a systematic review and dose-response meta-analysis of prospective studies. International Journal of Epidemiology, 46(3), 1029-1056. https://doi.org/10.1093/ije/dyw319

vitamin C, vitamin A, and potassium, which support heart health, vision, and immune function. Furthermore, the high fiber content in fruits and vegetables can help regulate blood sugar levels, lower cholesterol, and promote a healthy weight.

Intermittent Fasting Schedule

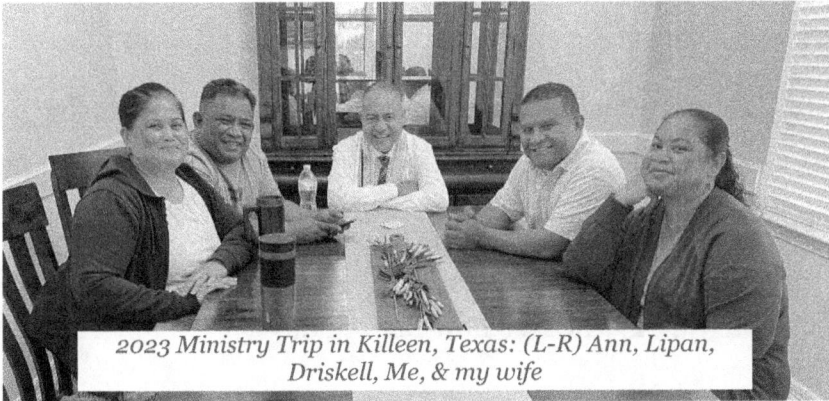

2023 Ministry Trip in Killeen, Texas: (L-R) Ann, Lipan, Driskell, Me, & my wife

Intermittent fasting (IF) is a dietary strategy involving periodic eating and fasting cycles. Some IF methods are time-restricted feeding, alternate-day fasting, and 5:2.[75] This eating pattern has gained popularity recently due to its potential health benefits, such as weight loss, improved metabolic health, and a reduced risk of chronic diseases.

Time-restricted feeding involves limiting daily food intake to a specific window, typically 6 to 10 hours, followed by a

[75] Patterson, R. E., & Sears, D. D. (2017). Metabolic Effects of Intermittent Fasting. Annual Review of Nutrition, 37, 371-393. https://doi.org/10.1146/annurev-nutr-071816-064634

fasting period of 14 to 18 hours. This method can be adapted to suit individual preferences and schedules, allowing for flexibility in meal planning.

Alternate-day fasting involves alternating between fasting days and eating days. On fasting days, calorie intake is significantly reduced, usually to about 25% of daily needs, while on eating days, regular food consumption is allowed.

The 5:2 method entails consuming a regular diet five days a week and then reducing calorie intake to about 25% of daily needs on the remaining two days. This approach may be more manageable for some individuals, allowing for greater freedom during the five non-fasting days.

Research has revealed that intermittent fasting can provide various health advantages, such as weight loss, better insulin sensitivity, and decreased inflammation.[76] Nevertheless, seeking guidance from a healthcare professional before initiating any new dietary plan is crucial, particularly for men aged 50 and above who might have pre-existing medical conditions or concerns.

Incorporating protein sources, whole grains, fruits, and vegetables into meals can significantly contribute to the

---

[76] de Cabo, R., & Mattson, M. P. (2019). Effects of Intermittent Fasting on Health, Aging, and Disease. The New England Journal of Medicine, 381(26), 2541-2551. https://doi.org/10.1056/NEJMra1905136

health and well-being of men over 50. These food groups provide essential nutrients that support muscle maintenance, weight management, and a reduced risk of chronic diseases. Alongside these dietary choices, intermittent fasting schedules can offer additional health benefits, such as weight loss, improved metabolic health, and reduced inflammation.

Before implementing any new dietary or fasting regimen, men over 50 must consult a healthcare professional to ensure that the chosen approach suits their needs and health status. By adopting a balanced diet and considering alternative eating patterns like intermittent fasting, men can support their overall health and well-being as they age.

Stay hydrated by drinking plenty of water.

Staying hydrated is critical to maintaining overall health and well-being, particularly for men over 50. Water is essential for various bodily functions, including digestion, absorption, transportation of nutrients, and regulation of body temperature.[77] Dehydration can result in various health issues, such as cognitive impairment, dizziness, and fatigue. Therefore, men aged 50 and above must consume sufficient daily water for proper hydration.

---

[77] Popkin, B. M., D'Anci, K. E., & Rosenberg, I. H. (2010). Water, hydration, and health. Nutrition Reviews, 68(8), 439-458. https://doi.org/10.1111/j.1753-4887.2010.00304.x

The water needed may vary depending on age, weight, physical activity level, and climate. Generally, consuming at least eight 8-ounce glasses of water per day is recommended. This amount may increase when engaging in regular physical activity or if living in a hot climate. Moreover, men 50 years and older should pay attention to their body's cues, such as the color of their urine and feelings of thirst, to determine whether they are consuming adequate water.

Control portion sizes and practice mindful eating.

As men age, their metabolism generally slows down, making it more challenging to sustain a healthy weight. One effective strategy for managing weight and promoting overall health is controlling portion sizes and adopting mindful eating practices. Mindful eating entails being attentive to hunger and satiety, savoring each bite, and fully engaging during meals.[78]

Controlling portion sizes can help prevent overeating and excessive calorie consumption, which can lead to weight gain. Men over 50 can use various techniques to control portion sizes, such as using smaller plates, serving food in individual

---

[78] Warren, J. M., Smith, N., & Ashwell, M. (2017). A structured literature review on the role of mindfulness, mindful eating and intuitive eating in changing eating behaviours: effectiveness and associated potential mechanisms. Nutrition Research Reviews, 30(2), 272–283. https://doi.org/10.1017/S0954422417000154

portions, and following the recommended sizes for different food groups.

Practicing mindful eating can also help men over 50 maintain a healthy weight and develop a better relationship with food. Mindful eating encourages listening to the body's hunger and fullness signals, eating slowly, and being present during meals. This practice can help prevent overeating, emotional eating, and binge eating, all of which can contribute to weight gain and poor health.

Try new foods and experiment with different recipes.

As men over 50 strive to maintain a healthy diet, it is essential to keep meals exciting and enjoyable by trying new foods and experimenting with different recipes. This approach can make healthy eating more appealing and ensure that men consume various nutrients to support their overall health.

Introducing new foods and recipes can help men over 50 discover new flavors, textures, and combinations they enjoy. This can also help expand their knowledge of different food groups and ingredients, making creating balanced, nutrient-dense meals easier.

Experimenting with different recipes can inspire men over

50 to find healthier alternatives to their favorite dishes. For example, they might try using whole-grain pasta instead of refined pasta, swapping sugary desserts for fruit-based treats, or incorporating more plant-based proteins. This can help men maintain a nutritious and enjoyable diet that supports their health and well-being as they age.

Staying hydrated by drinking plenty of water, controlling portion sizes, practicing mindful eating, and trying new foods and recipes are essential for men over 50 to maintain a healthy diet and promote overall well-being. By integrating these practices into their everyday routine, men can promote their well-being and savor a diverse and satisfying diet as they age.

Adopting a varied and nutritious diet is essential for men over 50 to ensure they receive the necessary nutrients to support their overall health and well-being. Men can maintain a healthy diet that promotes overall wellness by staying hydrated, controlling portion sizes, practicing mindful eating, and experimenting with new foods and recipes.

Proper hydration by drinking ample water is vital for various bodily functions, such as nutrient absorption, digestion, transportation, and body temperature regulation. Drinking at least eight glasses of water daily, each containing 8 ounces, can assist in preventing dehydration and the potential health problems associated with it.

Controlling portion sizes and practicing mindful eating can help men over 50 manage their weight and develop a better relationship with food. Mindful eating encourages listening to the body's hunger and fullness signals, eating slowly, and being present during meals, which can help prevent overeating, emotional eating, and binge eating.

Trying new foods and experimenting with different recipes can make healthy eating more enjoyable and ensure that men consume various nutrients. Introducing new foods and recipes can help men over 50 discover new flavors, textures, and combinations they enjoy while expanding their knowledge of different food groups and ingredients.

Incorporating these practices into their daily lives can help men over 50 support their health and enjoy a fulfilling and varied diet as they age. By staying focused on hydration, portion control, mindful eating, and trying new foods, men can continue to thrive in their later years and maintain a healthy and enjoyable lifestyle.

Talk to a nutritionist for additional guidance.

While adopting healthy eating habits is essential to maintaining overall health and well-being, men over 50 may also benefit from seeking additional guidance from a nutritionist. A nutritionist is a trained professional who can provide personalized advice and recommendations based on an individual's unique needs, health status, and dietary preferences.

Talking to a nutritionist can help men over 50 identify specific areas for improvement in their diet, set realistic goals, and develop a tailored plan to achieve those goals. Consulting a nutritionist can also offer direction on managing chronic health conditions such as diabetes, heart disease, or high blood pressure by implementing dietary modifications. Additionally, a nutritionist can offer valuable insights into the latest nutritional research and debunk common misconceptions about diet and health. They can help men over 50 navigate the often-confusing world of nutrition and make informed decisions about the foods they consume.

Men over 50 may also benefit from seeking guidance from a nutritionist if they have specific dietary concerns or requirements, such as food allergies, intolerances, or dietary restrictions. A nutritionist can help them plan a balanced and nutritious diet that accommodates these restrictions while providing all the necessary nutrients for optimal health. Talking to a nutritionist can be a valuable resource for men over 50 seeking to improve their diet and overall health. By seeking professional guidance, men can better understand their nutritional needs, develop a personalized plan for healthy eating, and receive support in managing any dietary challenges they may face.

Empowering Change Through Obesity Management and Nutrition

As we wrap up Chapter 2 on Obesity and Nutrition, let's take a moment to reflect on the key points we've navigated through in this complex yet vital topic. Our journey has underscored the importance of addressing obesity - a global health crisis that calls for immediate attention and proactive action.

We began by delving into the prevalence and causes of obesity, understanding the intricate interplay of genetic, environmental, and lifestyle factors. It became clear that obesity is not merely an individual issue; it's a societal challenge that requires comprehensive strategies to overcome.

We then unpacked the associated risks of obesity, such as cardiovascular diseases and type 2 diabetes. These conditions, along with the mental health implications of obesity, highlight the profound impact of this health crisis on individuals and communities alike.

This chapter's key area of focus was the importance of adopting a multi-faceted approach to addressing obesity. We explored strategies ranging from promoting healthy diets and increased physical activity to creating supportive environments and implementing policies that restrict the marketing of unhealthy foods.

Maintaining a healthy weight emerged as a crucial aspect of this discussion, with balanced nutrition, portion control, and mindful eating at its core. We also emphasized the benefits of regular exercise and physical activity for overall health and well-being.

Addressing obesity is not just about improving individual health outcomes; it's about enhancing the overall health of our communities and our world. As we conclude this chapter, our call to action is clear: Let's act today to positively change our lives and inspire others to do the same.

We can work towards a healthier future by implementing the strategies discussed in Chapter 2. This is not just an aspiration; it's a mission that demands our commitment and collective effort.

Let us embrace this challenge with determination and optimism, equipped with the knowledge we've gained and the tools we've been given. Together, we can turn the tide against obesity, improve individuals' and communities' overall health and well-being, and create a healthier future for all.

Key Points Checklist for Chapter 2: Obesity and Nutrition

1. **Comprehend Obesity's Scope**: Understand the definition, prevalence, and global impact of obesity on adults and children. Recognize obesity as a multifaceted health issue that requires our collective attention.
2. **Recognize the Causes**: Acknowledge the complex causes of obesity, including genetic and environmental factors. Understand that addressing obesity entails managing this intricate interplay of influences.
3. **Understand the Health Risks**: Be aware of the significant health risks associated with obesity, such as cardiovascular diseases, type 2 diabetes, certain cancers, and musculoskeletal disorders. Recognize that these risks extend beyond physical health, impacting mental well-being, too.
4. **Explore Management Strategies**: Learn about the diverse strategies for managing obesity. This includes embracing a healthy diet, increasing physical activity levels, and advocating for policy changes that support healthier lifestyles.
5. **Leverage Professional Guidance**: Seek guidance from healthcare professionals, like nutritionists, to develop tailored nutrition and exercise plans. Understand that everyone's journey with obesity is unique, and professional advice can be invaluable in navigating this path.

Call To Action:

Now that we've equipped ourselves with crucial knowledge about obesity, it's time to turn understanding into action. Let's commit to:

1. **Educate Ourselves and Others**: Share the knowledge you've gained about the causes and risks of obesity. Remember, education is the first step towards change.
2. **Adopt a Balanced Diet**: Embrace a nutritious diet rich in fruits, vegetables, whole grains, lean proteins, and healthy fats. Your body will thank you!
3. **Commit to Regular Exercise**: Aim for at least 150 minutes of moderate-intensity weekly exercise. Physical activity is a crucial ally in the fight against obesity.
4. **Seek Professional Guidance**: Reach out to healthcare professionals, like nutritionists, to develop personalized plans for nutrition and exercise. Their expertise can help you make the most of your health journey.
5. **Advocate for Healthy Policies**: Use your voice to advocate for policy changes that promote healthy environments and support individuals in making healthier lifestyle choices.

Remember, every step towards a healthier lifestyle is a step away from obesity. Let's rise to this challenge armed with knowledge, guided by professionals, and driven by a commitment to our health and the health of our communities. Together, we can make a difference!

Chapter 3: Promoting Active Lifestyle

"Physical fitness is not only one of the most important keys to a healthy body; it is the basis of dynamic and creative intellectual activity."

~ John F. Kennedy

As men get older, it becomes increasingly important to maintain an active lifestyle to promote optimal health and well-being. This is particularly relevant for men over 50, as this age group faces specific health challenges that can be managed and mitigated through regular physical activity, proper nutrition, and a focus on overall wellness.

Section A: Exercise Guidelines for Men Over 50

American College of Sports Medicine Exercise Guidelines

To maintain optimal health, men over 50 should strive to meet the American College of Sports Medicine's (ACSM) exercise guidelines (ACSM, 2018). These recommendations include engaging in at least 150 minutes of moderate-intensity aerobic exercise or 75 minutes of vigorous-intensity aerobic exercise per week and two or more days of strength training for all major muscle groups. These guidelines provide a strong foundation for men to pursue optimal health. Regular physical activity has been shown to provide numerous benefits, such as improving cardiovascular health, reducing the risk of chronic diseases, and promoting mental well-being.[79]

It is crucial to incorporate both aerobic and strength-training exercises into fitness routines. Aerobic exercises like walking, jogging, swimming, or cycling help improve cardiovascular fitness and endurance and contribute to weight management. On the other hand, strength training helps maintain muscle mass, which naturally declines with age and can improve balance, coordination, and overall functionality.[80]

It is also essential for men to consider flexibility and balance exercises, as these can help prevent age-related declines in mobility and reduce the risk of falling. Incorporating yoga, tai chi, or stretching routines into a

---

[79] Warburton, D. E., Nicol, C. W., & Bredin, S. S. (2006). Health benefits of physical activity: the evidence. *CMAJ : Canadian Medical Association journal = journal de l'Association medicale canadienne*, 174(6), 801–809. https://doi.org/10.1503/cmaj.051351

[80] Peterson, M. D., Rhea, M. R., & Alvar, B. A. (2005). Applications of the dose-response for muscular strength development: a review of meta-analytic efficacy and reliability for designing training prescription. *Journal of strength and conditioning research*, 19(4), 950–958. https://doi.org/10.1519/R-16874.1

weekly exercise regimen can enhance flexibility and balance.

However, men over 50 should remember to listen to their bodies and adjust their exercise routines accordingly. As we age, our bodies may require more time to recover from workouts, so it is essential to prioritize rest and recovery to prevent injuries and optimize performance.

The ACSM exercise guidelines can be followed if you strive for optimal health and fitness routines, including aerobics, strength, and flexibility. Older men can maintain and even improve their physical and mental health, leading to a better quality of life.

Prioritizing Strength and Balance Training for Enhanced Physical Performance:

Emphasizing strength and balance training is crucial to maintaining muscle mass, minimizing injury risk, and optimizing overall physical performance. A well-rounded fitness program should include a variety of exercises tailored to address these needs. Weightlifting, for instance, can help preserve and build muscle strength, while resistance bands offer adaptable and portable options for targeted muscle group training.

Bodyweight exercises, such as push-ups, squats, and lunges, provide an accessible and efficient way to develop strength using one's own body mass. Additionally, functional movements, like single-leg deadlifts or standing shoulder presses, can challenge the body's stability and coordination, improving balance and reducing the risk of falling. By focusing on strength and balance training, men over 50 can enjoy an active lifestyle with reduced injury risk and improved physical performance, paving the way for better overall health and well-being.

Embracing Challenging Exercises to Elevate Fitness Levels:

Men over 50 should strive to choose exercises that push their physical boundaries, allowing them to maintain and enhance their fitness levels. By incorporating challenging activities into their exercise routines, older adults can foster continued growth and improvements in their overall health.

Running, cycling, and swimming offer excellent opportunities to build cardiovascular endurance, vital for heart health and maintaining stamina for daily tasks. These aerobic exercises also help promote weight management and contribute to a positive mental state.

Resistance training is another essential component of a challenging fitness routine for men over 50. Incorporating exercises targeting various muscle groups, such as deadlifts, squats, and bench presses, can increase muscle strength and improve flexibility. Greater muscle strength and flexibility can translate into better balance and mobility, reducing the risk of falls and enhancing overall functionality.

Engaging in challenging exercises can also foster a sense of accomplishment and personal growth. As men over 50 continue to push their physical limits, they may find renewed motivation and a stronger sense of self-efficacy, contributing to an improved quality of life.

By embracing challenging exercises and striving for progress, men over 50 can enjoy the multiple benefits of an active lifestyle, including better cardiovascular health, increased muscle strength, and improved flexibility, leading to a more vibrant and fulfilling life experience.

Discovering the Power of Flexibility and Relaxation Exercises for Men over 50:

Men over 50 can significantly benefit from incorporating flexibility and relaxation exercises into their fitness routines, opening a world of improved physical and mental well-being. Practices such as yoga and tai chi offer a refreshing and enjoyable exercise approach, enhancing physical health and fostering inner peace and tranquility.

Yoga, an ancient practice with many styles, can be adapted

to suit any fitness level or personal preference. Its combination of stretching, strength-building, and mindfulness can help improve flexibility, balance, and posture. Regular yoga can also reduce stress levels, increase focus, and promote a positive mindset.

Tai chi, a gentle form of Chinese martial art, emphasizes slow, deliberate movements that harmonize the body and mind. As a low-impact practice, tai chi is an excellent choice for men over 50, as it can be easily adapted to accommodate individual needs. Regular tai chi practice can lead to an increased range of motion, better balance, and a reduced risk of falling. Additionally, the meditative nature of tai chi promotes relaxation and mental clarity, helping to manage stress and enhance overall well-being.

By exploring the world of flexibility and relaxation exercises, men over 50 can unlock a myriad of physical and mental benefits. By combining these practices with more traditional forms of exercise, older adults can achieve a holistic approach to fitness, leading to a more vibrant, balanced, and fulfilling lifestyle.

Embracing Low-Impact Activities for a Healthy, Active Lifestyle:

Low-impact activities offer an excellent alternative to more demanding exercises for men over 50 who may be experiencing joint pain or other physical limitations. These gentler forms of exercise can still deliver substantial health benefits while minimizing the risk of injury, allowing older adults to enjoy a healthy, active lifestyle without compromising their well-being.

Walking, for instance, is a simple yet powerful form of exercise that can be easily incorporated into daily life. Whether a leisurely stroll in the park or a brisk walk around the neighborhood, walking offers an accessible way to improve cardiovascular health, manage weight, and even boost mood. The social aspect of walking with friends or joining a walking group can also contribute to a greater sense of connection and camaraderie, further enhancing mental well-being.

Swimming is another low-impact activity that offers a full-body workout without stressing the joints. The buoyancy of water provides a supportive environment for exercise, reducing the impact on the body while allowing for an effective cardiovascular and strength-building workout. Swimming can improve muscle tone, flexibility, and endurance, all while providing a sense of relaxation and enjoyment. Cycling on a stationary bike or outdoors is yet another low-impact option for men over 50 looking to maintain their fitness. This activity can help build cardiovascular endurance, strengthen leg muscles, and improve balance and coordination. Cycling can also be a fun and social activity, with group rides or scenic routes providing opportunities for exploration and connection with others.

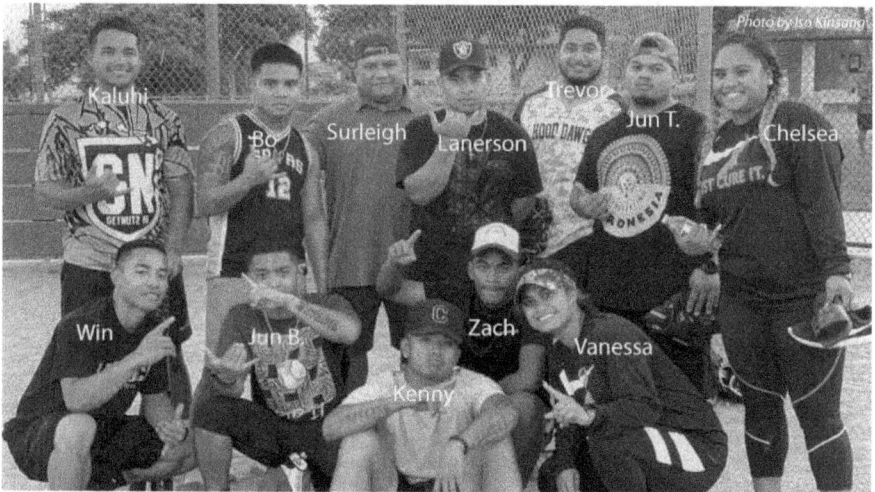

2021 San Diego California Softball Tournament with Youngins

By incorporating low-impact activities into their fitness routines, people over the age of fifty can enjoy the numerous health benefits of exercise without putting undue strain on their joints or exacerbating existing physical limitations. By finding activities that are both enjoyable and accessible, older adults can cultivate a sustainable, engaging approach to fitness that supports a healthy, active lifestyle well into their later years.

Honoring Your Body and Embracing Rest for Sustainable Fitness:

For men over 50, it is vital to recognize and respond to their bodies' signals. This is an essential part of maintaining a healthy, active lifestyle. By listening to the body's cues and taking breaks, when necessary, older adults can create a more sustainable and enjoyable fitness journey that supports their well-being for years. Rest days into an exercise regimen allow the body to recover and repair itself. Giving the body time to heal can prevent overtraining and reduce the risk of injury, ultimately leading to better overall performance and progress. Rest days also offer an opportunity to focus on other aspects of well-being, such as mental health or spending quality time with friends and family. Modifying exercises to accommodate physical limitations is another crucial aspect of listening to one's body. For example, if joint pain makes traditional squats difficult, a modified version using a chair for support can still offer strength-building benefits without causing discomfort.

By adjusting and choosing alternative exercises, men over 50 can continue to reap the rewards of physical activity while respecting their bodies' unique needs and limitations. Additionally, staying in tune with one's body also involves recognizing signs of fatigue, dehydration, or other discomforts during exercise. By taking breaks when needed or adjusting the intensity of a workout, older adults can ensure that their exercise routine remains safe and enjoyable.

By listening to their bodies and embracing rest, men over 50 can create a balanced and engaging approach to fitness that supports their physical and emotional well-being. Honoring the body's needs and adjusting as needed can lead to enjoying a fulfilling, active lifestyle throughout the later years.

The Importance of Consulting Healthcare Professionals for Personalized Fitness Guidance:

Before embarking on any new exercise program, men over 50 must consult a healthcare professional. By doing so, they can ensure that the chosen activities align with their unique health needs and goals, minimizing potential risks and optimizing the benefits of their fitness journey.

Healthcare professionals, such as primary care physicians, physiotherapists, or registered dietitians, can provide valuable insights into the most appropriate forms of exercise for everyone.[81] These experts can assess an individual's medical history, fitness level, and pre-existing conditions or limitations. Healthcare professionals can provide personalized exercise types, intensity levels, and frequency

Liguori, G., & American College of Sports Medicine. (2020). *ACSM's guidelines for exercise testing and prescription.* Lippincott Williams & Wilkins.

recommendations by considering these factors. Seeking guidance from a healthcare professional can also help men over 50 set realistic and achievable fitness goals. These experts can provide evidence-based advice on progressing safely and effectively, ensuring that individuals are challenged without risking their health.

Section B: Nutrition Tips for Healthy Eating:

Achieving a Balanced Diet for Optimal Health:

As men reach the age of fifty and beyond, it becomes increasingly important to prioritize a balanced diet that supports overall health and well-being. By incorporating diverse, nutrient-rich foods, older adults can provide their bodies with the essential fuel needed for daily activities and optimal health.

- Fruits and Vegetables: A diet rich in fruits and vegetables is crucial for men over 50, as they provide essential vitamins, minerals, and antioxidants. These nutrients support immune function and heart health and can help prevent chronic diseases such as diabetes and cancer. Aim to consume a colorful variety of fruits and vegetables daily, as different colors indicate different nutrients.

- Whole Grains: Whole grains, such as brown rice, quinoa, whole wheat bread, and oats, provide complex carbohydrates, fiber, and essential vitamins and minerals. These foods can help maintain steady energy levels, support digestive health, and contribute to healthy weight management.

- Lean Proteins: Consuming lean proteins, such as poultry, fish, beans, and legumes, is vital for muscle maintenance and recovery, particularly for men engaging in regular physical activity. These protein sources also supply essential amino acids, which the body cannot produce independently and must obtain through diet.

- Healthy Fats: Incorporating healthy fats into the diet, such as those found in avocados, nuts, seeds, and olive oil, is crucial for supporting brain health, hormone regulation, and reducing inflammation. These fats can also help improve heart health by promoting healthy cholesterol levels.

- Hydration: Staying well hydrated is essential for men over 50, as it supports various bodily functions, including digestion, temperature regulation, and joint lubrication. Drinking enough water throughout the day can also aid in appetite control and prevent dehydration, negatively impacting energy levels and cognitive function.

Men over 50 can support their overall health, well-being, and longevity by focusing on a balanced diet that includes various nutrient-dense foods. This approach to nutrition can also enhance the effectiveness of their exercise routines, ensuring they have the energy and nutrients necessary to maintain an active lifestyle.

The Importance of Limiting Processed Foods and Sugar-Sweetened Beverages:

Prioritizing a diet rich in whole, unprocessed foods and limiting the consumption of processed foods and sugar-sweetened beverages can play a significant role in maintaining optimal health and preventing chronic health conditions. It is not only crucial in your fifties but also in your younger days for your overall well-being.

A. **Processed Foods:** Processed foods often contain high levels of unhealthy fats, sodium, and added sugars. These ingredients can contribute to weight gain, increased blood pressure, and elevated cholesterol levels, increasing the risk of developing heart disease, type 2 diabetes, and other chronic conditions. Moreover, processed foods are low in essential nutrients, fiber, and antioxidants, crucial for maintaining overall health and well-being.

When men over 50 focus on whole, unprocessed foods, they provide their bodies with the nutrients needed to support a healthy lifestyle while avoiding the harmful effects of processed foods.

B. **Sugar-Sweetened Beverages:** Sugar-sweetened beverages, such as sodas, energy drinks, and sweetened fruit juices, are a significant source of added sugars. Consuming these beverages can lead to weight gain, an increased risk of type 2 diabetes, and dental issues such as tooth decay.

Additionally, sugar-sweetened beverages can contribute to inflammation in the body, which may exacerbate existing health conditions or increase the risk of developing chronic diseases. Replacing these beverages with healthier alternatives, such as water, herbal teas, or unsweetened beverages, can help men over 50 maintain a healthier diet and reduce the risk of chronic health issues. Now that they make conscious choices to consume whole, nutrient-dense foods and limit unhealthy options, older adults can better manage their weight, reduce the risk of chronic diseases, and support a vibrant, active lifestyle.

Low-Fat Dairy Products for Bone Health:

Incorporating low-fat dairy products into the diet can provide essential nutrients such as calcium and vitamin D, essential for maintaining bone health, particularly as men age.[82] These nutrients are crucial for supporting bone density, reducing the risk of fractures, and promoting overall skeletal health. Some low-fat dairy products include low-fat milk, yogurt, and cheese.

In addition to dairy products, non-dairy sources of calcium and vitamin D can also benefit those who may be lactose intolerant or prefer plant-based alternatives. Foods such as fortified plant-based milk, tofu, and leafy greens are excellent sources of calcium, while vitamin D can be obtained from sunlight exposure and fortified foods.

Limiting Red and Processed Meats for Overall Health:

Consuming excessive amounts of red and processed meats

---

[82] US, D. (2004). Bone health and osteoporosis: A Report of the Surgeon General. *http://www. surgeongeneral. gov/library/bonehealth/content. html.*

can increase the risk of heart disease and certain types of cancer, such as colorectal cancer.[83] These meats are often high in saturated fats and cholesterol, which can contribute to the development of atherosclerosis and other cardiovascular issues. Processed meats can contain high levels of sodium and preservatives, which may further increase health risks.

By limiting the consumption of red and processed meats and opting for leaner protein sources, such as poultry, fish, beans, and legumes, men over 50 can support their overall health and reduce the risk of chronic diseases. Additionally, incorporating plant-based protein sources can offer a variety of nutrients and health benefits, further promoting a well-rounded, balanced diet.

Opting for Lean Protein Sources and Supporting Muscle Mass:

Men over 50 should limit their high-fat and processed meats intake instead of lean protein sources such as poultry, fish and plant-based options like beans and legumes to maintain overall health and support muscle mass. A diverse range of protein sources can provide the amino acids required for muscle repair, recovery, and growth.

Bouvard, V., Loomis, D., Guyton, K. Z., Grosse, Y., El Ghissassi, F., Benbrahim-Tallaa, L., ... & Straif, K. (2015). Carcinogenicity of consumption of red and processed meat. *The Lancet Oncology*, 16(16), 1599–1600.

For optimal health, men should consume approximately 0.8 grams of protein per kilogram of body weight each day.[84] This can be achieved by combining animal and plant-based protein sources, ensuring a balanced diet that supports muscle maintenance and overall well-being.

The Benefits of Omega-3 Fatty Acids:

Incorporating foods rich in omega-3 fatty acids, such as salmon, walnuts, and chia seeds, can provide numerous health benefits for men over 50. Omega-3 fatty acids have been shown to improve cardiovascular health by reducing blood pressure, lowering triglycerides, and preventing the formation of arterial plaques (Mozaffarian & Wu, 2011). Additionally, these essential fatty acids have been linked to reduced inflammation in the body, which can help alleviate joint pain and stiffness often experienced by older adults.

The Importance of Choosing Unsaturated Vegetable Oils:

Making healthier choices regarding dietary fats is crucial for maintaining heart health and supporting overall well-being. Unsaturated vegetable oils, such as olive, avocado, and

---

[84] Rodriguez, N. R., DiMarco, N. M., & Langley, S. (2009). Position of the American Dietetic Association, Dietitians of Canada, and the American College of Sports Medicine: Nutrition and athletic performance. *Journal of the American Dietetic Association*, 109(3), 509–527.

canola oil, offer numerous health benefits compared to saturated fats like butter or lard.

A. **Improved Heart Health:** Unsaturated fats, mainly monounsaturated fats found in olive and avocado oils, have been shown to help lower LDL (low-density lipoprotein) cholesterol, often called *bad* cholesterol. By reducing LDL levels, these fats contribute to a lower risk of heart disease and stroke.

B. **Reduced Inflammation:** Unsaturated fats have been associated with reduced inflammation in the body. Chronic inflammation is linked to various health issues, including arthritis, diabetes, and heart disease. Consuming unsaturated fats instead of saturated fats can help decrease inflammation and support overall health.

C. **Weight Management:** Although all fats provide the same number of calories per gram, unsaturated fats may have a more favorable impact on weight management than saturated fats. Studies have suggested that consuming unsaturated fats can help promote feelings of fullness and maintain a healthy weight.[85]

D. **Enhanced Nutrient Absorption:** Unsaturated fats can aid in absorbing fat-soluble vitamins, such as vitamins A, D, E, and K. Incorporating healthy fats into the diet can ensure that the body receives and utilizes these essential nutrients effectively.

Monitoring Portion Sizes and Limiting Added Sugars, Sodium, and Saturated Fat:

Be mindful of portion sizes and limit your added sugars, sodium, and saturated fat intake. This can help to prevent weight gain, support heart health, and reduce the risk of chronic diseases.

[85] Paniagua, J. A., Gallego de la Sacristana, A., Romero, I., Vidal-Puig, A., Latre, J. M., Sanchez, E., Perez-Martinez, P., Lopez-Miranda, J., & Perez-Jimenez, F. (2007). Monounsaturated fat-rich diet prevents central body fat distribution and decreases postprandial adiponectin expression induced by a carbohydrate-rich diet in insulin-resistant subjects. *Diabetes care*, 30(7), 1717–1723. https://doi.org/10.2337/dc06-2220

Section C: Physical Activity and Its Role in Maintaining Optimal Health

Maintaining Muscle Strength, Flexibility, and Balance:

Regular physical activity is essential for men over 50 to maintain muscle strength, flexibility, and balance.

Muscle mass tends to decline as men age, leading to decreased strength and mobility. A consistent exercise routine that includes strength training, aerobic exercise, and flexibility-focused activities, such as yoga or tai chi, can help counteract these age-related changes and maintain overall functionality and independence.

Improving Mood and Reducing Stress:

Physical activity has been shown to improve mood and reduce stress levels by increasing the production of endorphins, the brain's natural *feel-good* chemicals.[86] Regular exercise can contribute to a better quality of life for men over 50 by helping to alleviate anxiety, depression, and stress, ultimately promoting emotional well-being.

---

[86] Mandolesi, L., Polverino, A., Montuori, S., Foti, F., Ferraioli, G., Sorrentino, P., & Sorrentino, G. (2018). Effects of Physical Exercise on Cognitive Functioning and Wellbeing: Biological and Psychological Benefits. *Frontiers in psychology*, 9, 509. https://doi.org/10.3389/fpsyg.2018.00509

Enhancing Cardiovascular Health:

Regular exercise can help lower the risk of heart disease by improving cardiovascular health and promoting healthy blood flow. Physical activity has been linked to reduced blood pressure, improved cholesterol levels, and better glucose control, all contributing to a lower risk of developing cardiovascular issues.

Improving Sleep Quality:

Physical activity can improve sleep quality by helping regulate the body's circadian rhythm and promoting relaxation.[87] Adequate sleep is essential for overall health and well-being, allowing the body to recover, repair, and maintain cognitive function. Regular exercise can help men over 50 achieve better sleep quality and, in turn, support their overall health.

Strengthening Bones and Joints

Weight-bearing exercises and strength training can help strengthen bones and joints, reducing the risk of osteoporosis and age-related joint issues. By maintaining strong bones and joints, men over 50 can prevent fractures and maintain their

---

[87] Kredlow, M. A., Capozzoli, M. C., Hearon, B. A., Calkins, A. W., & Otto, M. W. (2015). The effects of physical activity on sleep: a meta-analytic review. *Journal of behavioral medicine*, 38(3), 427–449. https://doi.org/10.1007/s10865-015-9617-6

mobility, independence, and quality of life.

Reducing the Risk of Chronic Illnesses:

Regular physical activity can help reduce the risk of chronic illnesses such as obesity, diabetes, and certain types of cancer. Exercise can help maintain a healthy weight, regulate blood sugar levels, and boost the immune system, all contributing to a decreased risk of developing chronic health conditions.

Increasing Mental Alertness and Cognitive Function:

Physical activity has increased mental alertness and cognitive function, which can be particularly beneficial for men over 50 as they face age-related cognitive decline. Exercise can improve memory, sharpen concentration, and enhance problem-solving abilities, enabling men to stay mentally sharp and engaged as they age.

Enhancing Social Connections:

Physical activity can provide opportunities for social connections, helping to reduce feelings of isolation or loneliness that older men may experience. Group activities, such as sports leagues, exercise classes, or walking clubs, can foster camaraderie and support networks, contributing to a greater sense of belonging and improved mental health.

Adopting an active lifestyle is crucial for men over 50 to promote optimal health and maintain a high quality of life. By following the exercise guidelines, adhering to a balanced diet, and recognizing the many benefits of physical activity, men in this age group can effectively manage age-related health challenges and thrive in their later years. By taking a proactive approach to fitness, nutrition, and overall wellness, men can enjoy greater vitality, longevity, and happiness as they navigate their golden years.

Key Points Checklist for Chapter 3: Promoting Active Lifestyle

1. **Understand Exercise Guidelines for Men Over 50**: Acknowledge the specific exercise requirements for men over 50. This includes a balanced mix of aerobic exercises, strength training, and flexibility exercises to maintain fitness and overall health.

2. **Prioritize Strength and Balance Training**: Recognize the importance of strength and balance training in maintaining muscle mass, reducing injury risk, and optimizing physical performance. Remember, aging doesn't mean slowing down; it's about adapting and staying strong!

3. **Embrace Challenging Exercises**: Increase your fitness levels by incorporating challenging exercises into your routine. These will improve your physical health and keep you mentally sharp and energized.

4. **Discover Flexibility and Relaxation Exercises**: Explore the benefits of yoga and tai chi, among other exercises. These activities enhance your physical flexibility and mental well-being, promoting a sense of calm and relaxation.

5. **Incorporate Low-Impact Activities**: Engage in low-impact activities like walking, swimming, or cycling. These are excellent ways to stay active and fit while minimizing strain on your joints, making them perfect for those over 50.

Call to Action:

Now that we've explored the key aspects of promoting an active lifestyle, particularly for men over 50, it's time to implement this knowledge. Here's your five-step action plan:

1. **Consult a Healthcare Professional**: Begin your fitness journey with professional advice. They can help tailor a fitness regimen that aligns with your unique health needs and goals, ensuring you get the most out of your efforts.

2. **Balance Your Diet**: Complement your active lifestyle with a nutritious diet. Add fruits, vegetables, whole grains, lean proteins, and healthy fats to your meals for optimal nutrition.

3. **Limit Unhealthy Foods**: Reduce your intake of processed foods, sugar-sweetened beverages, and red/processed meats. These small changes can significantly lower your risk of chronic health conditions.

4. **Monitor Your Portion Sizes**: Monitor portion sizes and limit added sugars, sodium, and saturated fats. This will aid in weight management and promote heart health.

5. **Stay Active Regularly**: Make physical activity a part of your daily routine. Whether it's strength training, aerobic exercises, or low-impact activities, remember that consistency is vital to maintaining muscle strength, improving cardiovascular health, and enhancing mood.

The journey to an active lifestyle is personal and filled with challenges and triumphs. But remember, each step you take towards a healthier lifestyle is a step towards improved well-being, enhanced quality of life, and reduced risk of chronic illnesses. So, let's get moving and embrace the power of an active lifestyle!

Chapter 4: Preventative Measures

"True prevention is not waiting for bad things to happen; it's preventing things from happening in the first place."

~ Don McPherson

Preventative screenings are crucial to maintaining optimal health, especially for men over 50, as they can help detect and address health issues early on. Prostate cancer is a commonly diagnosed cancer among men and is regarded as the second most frequent cause of cancer-related fatalities in men in the United States.[88]

Detecting prostate cancer early is crucial for improving treatment outcomes and survival rates. Regular prostate exams, including the Digital Rectal Exam (DRE) and the Prostate-Specific Antigen (PSA) test, are essential for the early detection and management of prostate cancer.

Aside from getting screened for prostate cancer, men over 50 should also undergo regular health screenings, including blood pressure checks, cholesterol tests, and colonoscopies, to

---

[88] American Cancer Society. (2021). Key statistics for prostate cancer. Retrieved from https://www.cancer.org/cancer/prostate-cancer/about/key-statistics.html

ensure the proper monitoring and maintenance of their overall health. Age-appropriate vaccinations and lifestyle modifications, such as exercise and a healthy diet, can further contribute to a longer and healthier life. This chapter will discuss the importance of preventative screenings for men over 50, focusing on prostate exams. The aim is to raise awareness about the need for regular screenings and their role in the early detection and prevention of health issues.

By understanding the significance of these tests and overcoming potential barriers to accessing them, men can take charge of their health and ensure their well-being as they age.

Overview of Prostate Exams

Digital Rectal Exam (DRE)

The Digital Rectal Exam (DRE) is a simple and quick procedure where a healthcare professional inserts a gloved, lubricated finger into the patient's rectum to assess the size, shape, and texture of the prostate gland. This examination can help identify any abnormalities or changes in the prostate that may indicate the presence of cancer or other conditions.

Although the DRE may be uncomfortable, it is generally not painful and usually takes less than a minute to perform.

Regular DREs can contribute to the early detection of prostate cancer, increasing the chances of successful treatment.

The importance of the DRE as a screening tool should not be underestimated. Despite its invasive nature, it is often the first step in detecting potential prostate issues. The DRE allows healthcare providers to detect irregularities, such as lumps, nodules, or hardness in the prostate gland, which may indicate cancer or other prostate conditions.

In some cases, the DRE may be the only method to detect these abnormalities, as the PSA test may not always show elevated levels in the presence of cancer.

The DRE has some limitations, as it can only assess the part of the prostate gland closest to the rectal wall. Additionally, the examination relies on the healthcare provider's expertise in conducting the exam, which may result in variations in accuracy.

Despite these limitations, the DRE remains a vital component of prostate cancer screening and is often used with the PSA test to improve detection rates.

Baseline PSA Screening

The recommendation for Prostate-Specific Antigen (PSA) screening for healthy men, including veterans, has been debated. In the past, PSA screening fell out of favor due to professional guidelines based on short-term trial results, including the PLCO Cancer Screening Trial, which was later identified as having faulty data.[89] However, recent studies suggest that the benefits of PSA screening outweigh its potential harms, emphasizing the need for a resurgence in screening rates.[90]

Veterans, in particular, should be considered for routine PSA screening due to their unique health profiles and potential exposure to various environmental hazards during service. A study conducted among veterans found an association between lower PSA screening rates and increased incidents of metastatic prostate cancer, further underlining the importance of regular screening.[91]

Despite the growing body of evidence supporting PSA screening, there is a clear need for straightforward messaging and guidance from expert panels to ensure that men are not left in confusion. Shared decision-making, a process where healthcare providers and patients work together to select

---

[89] Shoag JE, Mittal S, Hu JC. Reevaluating PSA testing rates in the PLCO trial. N Engl J Med. 2016;374(18):1795-1796.

[90] Shoag JE, Nyame YA, Gulati R, Etzioni R, Hu JC. Reconsidering the trade-offs of prostate cancer screening. N Engl J Med. 2020;382(25):2465-2468.

[91] Bryant AK, Lee KM, Alba PR, et al. Association of prostate-specific antigen screening rates with subsequent metastatic prostate cancer incidence at US Veterans Health Administration facilities. JAMA Oncol. 2022;8(12):1747-1755.

tests, treatments, or care plans, is also crucial in this context.[92,93]

Moreover, the potential use of MRI as a triage test and active surveillance for indolent cancer can help tailor the approach to everyone's risk profile, thus improving outcomes (Donovan et al., 2016; Donovan et al., 2023).[94, 95]

The call for clear guidance on baseline PSA screening for healthy men, including veterans, has never been more urgent. It's time to move beyond ambiguity and embrace a proactive approach towards preventative measures.

Transrectal Ultrasound (TRUS)

Transrectal ultrasound (TRUS) is another imaging technique used to evaluate the prostate gland, particularly in cases where abnormalities are detected through a DRE or elevated PSA levels. Transrectal ultrasound (TRUS) is a

---

[92] Légaré F, Ratte S, Gravel K, Graham ID. Barriers and facilitators to implementing shared decision-making in clinical practice: update of a systematic review of health professionals' perceptions. Patient Educ Couns. 2008;73(3):526-535.

[93] Jiang C, Fedewa SA, Wen Y, Jemal A, Han X. Shared decision making and prostate-specific antigen based prostate cancer screening following the 2018 update of USPSTF screening guideline. Prostate Cancer Prostatic Dis. 2021;24(1):77-80.

[94] Donovan JL, Hamdy FC, Lane JA, et al. Patient-reported outcomes after monitoring, surgery, or radiotherapy for prostate cancer. N Engl J Med. 2016;375(15):1425-1437.

[95] Donovan JL, Hamdy FC, Lane JA, et al. Patient-reported outcomes 12 years after localized prostate cancer treatment. NEJM Evid. 2023;10.1056/EVIDoa2300018.

medical imaging technique that uses sound waves to produce visual representations of the prostate.

This procedure provides healthcare providers with significant insights into the gland's size, shape, and structure, enabling them to make informed decisions regarding diagnosis and treatment.[96]

This non-invasive procedure can help identify potential issues with the prostate and guide further diagnostic tests and treatment options. During a TRUS procedure, a small ultrasound probe is inserted into the rectum, allowing for a detailed prostate gland examination. During a transrectal ultrasound (TRUS), a specialized probe emits sound waves that penetrate the prostate tissue and reflect, creating echoes. A computer then converts these echoes into visual images, providing valuable information about the prostate's internal structure, including any abnormalities or potential issues that may require further investigation. These images can help healthcare providers identify any irregularities, such as masses, cysts, or areas of inflammation, that may require further investigation.

TRUS has several advantages over other prostate screening methods. It provides real-time prostate imaging, enabling

---

[96] Radiological Society of North America. (2021). Prostate/Transrectal Ultrasound. Retrieved from https://www.radiologyinfo.org/en/info/prostate-trus

healthcare providers to detect abnormalities that may not be identified through a DRE or PSA test alone. Additionally, TRUS can help estimate the size of the prostate gland, which can be useful in diagnosing conditions such as benign prostatic hyperplasia (BPH) or determining the extent of prostate cancer.

While TRUS offers valuable insights into prostate health, it is essential to note that it cannot definitively diagnose prostate cancer alone. In cases where TRUS reveals suspicious areas or lesions, a healthcare provider may recommend a prostate biopsy to obtain tissue samples for further analysis.

TRUS, or transrectal ultrasound-guided biopsy, is commonly used to collect prostate tissue samples. The real-time imaging capabilities of TRUS allow healthcare providers to accurately target suspicious areas, increasing the likelihood of obtaining a representative tissue sample.

Like any medical procedure, TRUS has some limitations and potential risks. Although it provides valuable information about the prostate gland, it may not always detect small or early-stage cancers. Furthermore, the procedure may cause some discomfort or pain, and there is a small risk of infection or bleeding associated with the insertion of the ultrasound probe.

Nevertheless, TRUS remains a crucial component of prostate cancer screening and diagnosis, particularly in cases where other screening methods reveal potential concerns.

Other Recommended Screening Tests for Men Over 50

Colon Cancer Screening

Colorectal or colon cancer can affect both men and women and is considered one of the most widespread forms of cancer. Sadly, it is also a leading cause of death among cancer patients.

Early detection of colon cancer through regular screening can significantly improve treatment outcomes and survival rates. For men over 50, it is recommended to undergo colon cancer screening, as the risk of developing this cancer increases with age.

There are several methods available for colon cancer screening, including:

Fecal Occult Blood Test (FOBT) or Fecal Immunochemical Test (FIT): These tests are specifically intended to find blood in the stool, which can indicate potential gastrointestinal conditions, such as colon cancer, in their early stages. The tests are non-invasive and can be done at home with a kit provided by a healthcare provider. If the results are positive, further testing, such as a colonoscopy, may be required to determine the cause of the bleeding.

Flexible Sigmoidoscopy: This procedure involves the insertion of a thin, flexible tube with a light and camera at the end into the rectum and lower colon to examine the lining for abnormalities, such as polyps or tumors. Flexible sigmoidoscopy does not require sedation and can be performed in a healthcare provider's office. A colonoscopy may be recommended for a more detailed examination if any abnormalities are found.

Colonoscopy: This is a more comprehensive examination of the colon and rectum. The process involves inserting a flexible tube with a light and camera attached to the end through the rectum and maneuvering it along the colon. A healthcare provider can detect and remove polyps or take tissue samples for further analysis during the colonoscopy. This procedure usually requires sedation and is performed in a healthcare facility.

Medical experts advise men at average risk of developing colon cancer to commence routine screenings at the age of forty-five. Screening options may include annual FOBT or FIT, flexible sigmoidoscopy every five years, or colonoscopy every ten years.[97]

People at an increased risk of developing colon cancer, for instance, those with a family history of colon cancer or inflammatory bowel disease, may need to undergo screening at an earlier age and more frequently than individuals with an Avera. This can help ensure that potential signs of colon cancer are identified as soon as possible, leading to more effective treatment and better outcomes.

Skin Cancer Screening

Skin cancer is the most frequently diagnosed among all types of cancer, and men aged fifty and above are more susceptible to this ailment. Early skin cancer detection, particularly melanoma, can significantly improve treatment outcomes and survival rates. Regular skin cancer screening can help identify abnormal skin growths, moles, or lesions that may require further examination or treatment.

There are two primary components of skin cancer screening:

    A. Self-examination: Men over 50 should perform monthly self-examinations of their skin to

---

[97] American Cancer Society. (2021). American Cancer Society Guideline for Colorectal Cancer Screening. Retrieved from https://www.cancer.org/cancer/colon-rectal-cancer/detection-diagnosis-staging/acs-recommendations.html

monitor for any changes in the appearance of moles, freckles, or other skin growths. They should look for the ABCDEs of melanoma—Asymmetry, Border irregularity, Color variation, Diameter more significant than a pencil eraser, and Evolving appearance (changes in size, shape, or color). If any suspicious changes are noticed, it is crucial to consult a healthcare provider for further evaluation.

B. Clinical skin examination: A healthcare provider, such as a dermatologist, can perform a thorough skin examination during routine checkups or upon request. They will evaluate any areas of concern and may take a biopsy of suspicious lesions for further analysis. It is essential to undergo regular clinical skin examinations for individuals at a higher risk of developing skin cancer, such as those with fair skin, a family history of skin cancer, or excessive sun exposure.

Men over 50 years of age may also benefit from such exams. By having their skin regularly checked by a healthcare professional, individuals can identify any suspicious moles or lesions at an early stage and seek prompt treatment if necessary.[98]

Men over 50 must prioritize regular colon and skin cancer screenings to maintain optimal health. Early detection and intervention are crucial in improving treatment outcomes and survival rates for both colon and skin cancer. By staying informed about screening options and recommendations, men can take proactive steps to protect their health and well-being.

Blood Pressure and Cholesterol Tests:

Regular blood pressure and cholesterol screenings are essential for men over 50, as they can help identify potential cardiovascular health issues. Elevated cholesterol levels and high blood pressure (hypertension) are two factors that can increase an individual's risk of developing severe health conditions, such as heart disease and stroke. It is essential to manage these conditions to reduce the risk of developing such complications.

A. **Blood Pressure:** Blood pressure is the pressure exerted by the blood against the artery walls as it is propelled by the heart throughout the body. Two

---

[98] American Cancer Society. (2021). Skin Cancer Prevention and Early Detection. Retrieved from https://www.cancer.org/cancer/skin-cancer/prevention-and-early-detection.html

numbers are measured to determine an individual's blood pressure: systolic pressure (the top number) and diastolic pressure (the bottom number). Men over 50 should undergo blood pressure checks at least once a year or more frequently if they have a history of hypertension or other risk factors. By regularly monitoring blood pressure, individuals can help identify any potential issues and take steps to manage them effectively.

B. **Cholesterol:** Cholesterol is a waxy substance found in the blood that is essential for the body to function correctly. Elevated levels of low-density lipoprotein (LDL) cholesterol, commonly known as *bad* cholesterol, can significantly enhance the risk of developing heart disease. Men over 50 should have their cholesterol levels checked every four to six years or more frequently if they have a history of high cholesterol or other risk factors.[99]

Diabetes Screening:

Diabetes is a chronic medical condition that can cause difficulty regulating blood sugar levels. The most prevalent

---

[99] American Heart Association. (2021). How to Help Prevent Heart Disease At Any Age. Retrieved from https://www.heart.org/en/healthy-living/healthy-lifestyle/how-to-help-prevent-heart-disease-at-any-age

type of diabetes is type 2, which is more common in men over 50. If left untreated, this condition can increase the risk of developing severe health complications such as heart disease, stroke, kidney disease, and other related ailments. Early detection of diabetes can help prevent or delay these complications through appropriate management and lifestyle changes. Screening for diabetes typically involves a blood test to measure the amount of glucose (sugar) in the blood. The most common tests used for diabetes screening are the fasting plasma glucose (FPG) test and the hemoglobin A1C test. The FPG test determines blood sugar levels following an overnight fast, whereas the A1C test calculates the average blood sugar levels over the previous three months.[100]

Men over 50 should discuss their risk factors for diabetes with their healthcare provider to determine the appropriate frequency of diabetes screening. Certain factors can increase an individual's risk of developing type 2 diabetes, including being overweight or obese, having a family history of diabetes, experiencing high blood pressure, and having elevated cholesterol levels. It is essential to be aware of these risk factors and take steps to manage them to help reduce the risk of developing diabetes.

---

[100] Centers for Disease Control and Prevention. (2020). Diabetes Tests. retrieved from https://www.cdc.gov/diabetes/basics/getting-tested.html

Men over 50 prioritize regular blood pressure, cholesterol, and diabetes screenings to maintain optimal health. Early detection and management of these conditions can help prevent or delay serious health complications and improve overall well-being.

Eye Test:

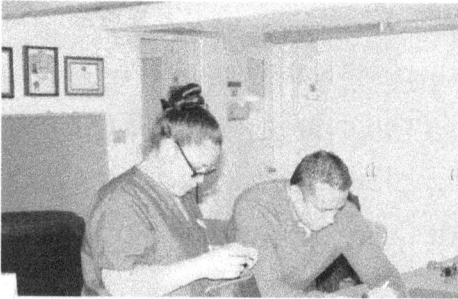

Dr. Asinech Hellan Pangelinan & her husband, Mike, providing optometry services.

Consistent eye examinations are paramount to preserving optimal vision and eye health, particularly for men aged fifty and above. With increasing age, the probability of experiencing age-related eye disorders, such as glaucoma, cataracts, and age-related macular degeneration, escalates. Early detection and appropriate management of these conditions can help preserve vision and prevent further complications. A comprehensive eye exam involves various tests to assess overall eye health and visual acuity. Some critical components of an eye exam include a visual acuity test, a dilated eye exam, and tonometry to measure eye pressure.[101] Men aged fifty and over should undergo a thorough eye examination at least once every two years. However, they may require more frequent eye exams if they have a history of eye problems or other risk factors.

Bone Density Evaluation:

Bone density evaluations, also known as bone mineral density (BMD) tests, measure the amount of calcium and other minerals in the bones to assess bone strength and fracture risk. As men age, the likelihood of developing osteoporosis, a condition that results in frail and fragile bones, rises. Consistent bone density assessments can aid in the early identification of bone loss and provide direction for suitable preventive arcs.

The most common method used for bone density evaluation is dual-energy X-ray absorptiometry (DXA), which uses low-dose X-rays to measure the spine, hip, or wrist BMD.[102] The results are presented in a T-score format after

---

[101] National Eye Institute. (2019). Get a Dilated Eye Exam. Retrieved from https://www.nei.nih.gov/learn-about-eye-health/healthy-vision/get-dilated-eye-exam
[102] National Osteoporosis Foundation. (n.d.). Bone Density Exam/Testing. Retrieved from https://www.nof.org/patients/diagnosis-information/bone-density-examtesting/

taking the bone mineral density (BMD) test. This score compares the individual's BMD with that of a healthy young adult. A lower T-score suggests a greater risk of fractures. It is essential to be aware of one's T-score and take appropriate measures to manage the risk of fractures, such as lifestyle changes or medication.

Men over 50 should discuss their risk factors for osteoporosis with their healthcare provider to determine the appropriate frequency of bone density evaluations. Risk factors for osteoporosis in men include a history of fractures, low body weight, the use of certain medications, and a family history of osteoporosis.

Men over 50 should prioritize regular eye exams and bone density evaluations to maintain optimal health. Early detection and appropriate management of age-related eye conditions and bone loss can help prevent complications and improve overall well-being.

Mental Health Check-up:

Mental health is essential to overall well-being, particularly for men over 50, who may experience unique stressors and challenges as they age. Mental health check-ups can help identify and address potential issues, such as depression, anxiety, or cognitive decline, and ensure that individuals receive the necessary support and resources to maintain their mental well-being. A mental health check-up typically involves conversing with a healthcare provider or mental health professional about an individual's emotional well-being, stress levels, and concerns. This conversation may cover various topics, such as sleep patterns, mood fluctuations, coping strategies, and social support networks.

Healthcare providers may also use screening tools or questionnaires to assess symptoms of depression, anxiety, or other mental health conditions.[103]

Men over 50 should discuss their mental health with their healthcare provider during routine check-ups or if they experience significant changes in mood, energy levels, or overall well-being. Early detection and intervention of mental health issues can improve treatment outcomes and enhance the quality of life.

Mental health checkups are vital to optimal health for men over 50. By addressing mental health concerns proactively, individuals can better manage stress, maintain emotional well-being, and navigate the challenges of aging with resilience and support.

---

[103] National Institute of Mental Health. (2021). Help for Mental Illnesses. Retrieved from https://www.nimh.nih.gov/health/find-help

Key Points Checklist for Chapter 4: Preventative Measures

1. **Prostate Cancer Screenings**: Recognize the importance of regular prostate exams, including the Digital Rectal Exam (DRE) and the Prostate-Specific Antigen (PSA) test, for early detection and management of prostate cancer in men over 50.

2. **Comprehensive Health Screenings**: Understand the necessity of regular health screenings, including blood pressure, cholesterol tests, colonoscopies, and eye exams, to monitor and maintain optimal health.

3. **Colon Cancer Screenings**: Acknowledge the significance of colon cancer screening methods such as Fecal Occult Blood Test (FOBT), Flexible Sigmoidoscopy, or Colonoscopy to detect and treat this disease at its earliest stage.

4. **Skin Cancer Screenings**: Grasp the value of regular skin cancer screenings, including self-examinations and clinical skin examinations, to detect abnormal skin growths or lesions that may require further evaluation or treatment.

5. **Regular Health Check-ups**: Prioritize regular screenings for blood pressure, cholesterol levels, diabetes, bone density, and mental health to identify and manage potential health issues and uphold overall well-being.

Call to Action:

Now that we've explored the vital preventative measures necessary for men over 50, it's time to implement this knowledge. Here's your five-step action plan:

1. **Schedule Regular Prostate Exams**: Don't delay your DRE and PSA test. These crucial exams are your first line of defense against prostate cancer.

2. **Undergo Comprehensive Health Screenings**: Make blood pressure checks, cholesterol tests, colonoscopies, and eye exams a part of your regular health regimen. Remember, proactive monitoring is vital to maintaining your health.

3. **Get Screened for Colon Cancer**: Utilize methods like FOBT, Flexible Sigmoidoscopy, or Colonoscopy to stay ahead of colon cancer. Early detection can significantly improve treatment outcomes.

4. **Perform Regular Skin Examinations**: Keep an eye on your skin, and don't hesitate to seek a clinical skin examination if you notice any abnormal growths or lesions. Your vigilance can save your life!

5. **Prioritize Regular Health Check-ups**: Stay on top of your health by scheduling regular screenings for blood pressure, cholesterol levels, diabetes, bone density, and mental health. Your well-being is worth the effort!

Preventative measures are a powerful tool in our healthcare arsenal. We can significantly enhance our health outcomes and well-being by staying proactive, vigilant, and informed. So, let's commit to this checklist, take charge of our health, and pave the way toward a healthier future! Remember, when it comes to your health, every step counts.

Chapter 5: Erectile Dysfunction

"Religion is the impotence of the human mind to deal with occurrences it cannot understand."

~ Karl Marx

Introduction to Erectile Dysfunction

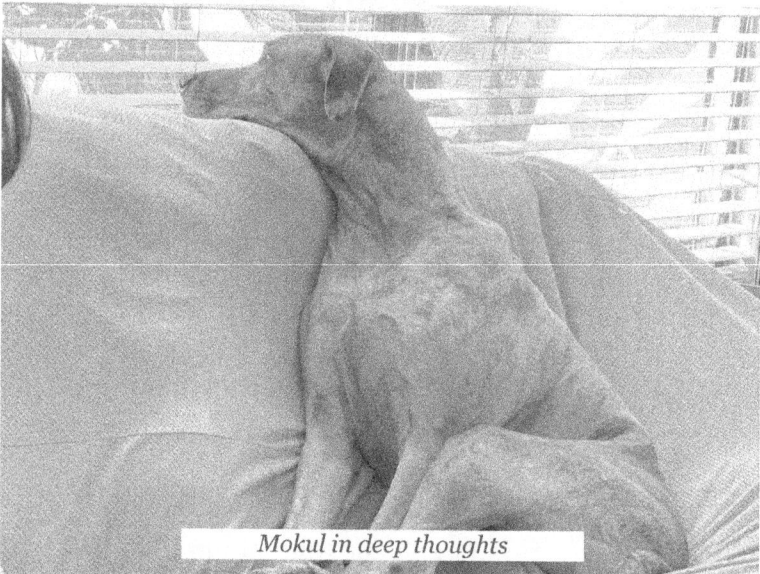
Mokul in deep thoughts

Welcome to a pivotal chapter in our exploration of men's health. In this section, we delve deep into an issue that has far-reaching implications for numerous men worldwide - Erectile Dysfunction (ED). This complex condition, often shrouded in misunderstanding and stigma, is more common than you might think and can significantly impact both physical health and emotional well-being.

Erectile Dysfunction, also known as impotence, is the persistent inability to achieve or maintain an erection sufficient for satisfactory sexual intercourse.[104] It's a challenge that doesn't discriminate by age, affecting men across all life stages.

While it's true that ED tends to become more prevalent as men age, it's not an inevitable part of growing older. Approximately 40% of men have experienced some form of ED by age 40. By the time they reach 70, that number rises to nearly 70%.[105] These figures underscore the widespread nature of this issue, one that every man should be aware of.

Beyond the physical manifestations, the effects of ED seep into all corners of a man's life. It can decrease sexual desire, create tension in relationships, and even result in stress, anxiety, and a decline in self-esteem. Further compounding

---

[104] Erectile Dysfunction, Mayo Clinic, Retrieved from: https://www.mayoclinic.org/diseases-conditions/erectile-dysfunction/symptoms-causes/syc-20355776

[105] Feldman HA, Goldstein I, Hatzichristou DG, Krane RJ, McKinlay JB. Impotence and its medical and psychosocial correlates: Results of the Massachusetts Male Aging Study. J Urol 1994; 151:54–61.

the issue, ED is often linked with other severe health conditions such as heart disease, diabetes, obesity, and high blood pressure.[106]

Moreover, lifestyle choices like smoking, alcohol consumption, and substance abuse can exacerbate the risk of developing ED. As such, understanding, evaluating, and treating ED are not just about improving sexual function – they are crucial steps toward enhancing overall health and well-being.

This chapter aims to shed light on Erectile Dysfunction, breaking down misconceptions and providing clear, actionable information. Because knowledge is power, and understanding ED is the first step towards a healthier, happier life.

Factors Contributing to Erectile Dysfunction

Genetic predispositions and their role in ED

In an unprecedented breakthrough, researchers have discovered a genetic variant near the SIM1 gene, which escalates the risk factor for Erectile Dysfunction (ED). This

---

[106] Population-level Prevalence, Scientific Report, Retrieved from: https://www.nature.com/articles/s41598-023-39968-9

condition impedes the capacity to achieve or maintain an erection suitable for satisfactory sexual activity. This discovery underscores the role of genetics in ED, supplementing our understanding that while the condition is more prevalent with age, aging itself is not the cause.[107]

The significance of this research lies in the revelation that the genetic variant can influence the functionality of the SIM1 gene, thereby contributing to ED. This insight, derived from a genome-wide association study, was corroborated in a second cohort of participants, solidifying its credibility. With this knowledge, we can develop targeted treatments to restore healthy sexual function by focusing on the SIM1 gene. This discovery is a scientific breakthrough and a beacon of hope for those affected by ED.[108]

Environmental factors leading to ED.

Erectile Dysfunction (ED), a condition marked by the consistent struggle to achieve or maintain an erection for satisfactory sexual activity, is not a consequence of aging alone. It's a complex issue with multiple contributing factors, including environmental influences and lifestyle choices. For

---

[107] Jorgenson E, Matharu N2, Palmer MR,...Van Den Eeden SK. Genetic variation in the SIM1 locus is associated with erectile dysfunction. NIH external link Proc Natl Acad Sci USA 115: 11018-11023, 2018.
[108] ipid.

instance, smoking, excessive alcohol consumption, and drug use can significantly increase the risk of developing ED.[109]

Smoking, in particular, damages blood vessels and obstructs the blood flow to the penis, thereby impeding the function of cells crucial for maintaining an erection. Similarly, excessive alcohol intake can upset hormonal balance, inflict liver damage, and impair nerves - all factors leading to ED. Furthermore, both prescription and illicit drugs can contribute to ED. Certain medications used to treat conditions like high blood pressure, depression, and anxiety can disrupt nerve signals and blood flow, making it challenging to achieve an erection. Recreational substances like cocaine and methamphetamine can also negatively impact sexual function. The good news is by making healthier lifestyle choices and avoiding substances known to harm sexual health; one can significantly reduce the risk of developing ED. Remember, your health is in your hands; every positive step can make a difference.

---

[109] Roychoudhury, Shubhadeep, Saptaparna Chakraborty, Arun Paul Choudhury, Anandan Das, Niraj Kumar Jha, Petr Slama, Monika Nath, Peter Massanyi, Janne Ruokolainen, and Kavindra Kumar Kesari. 2021. "Environmental Factors–Induced Oxidative Stress: Hormonal and Molecular Pathway Disruptions in Hypogonadism and Erectile Dysfunction" Antioxidants 10, no. 6: 837. https://doi.org/10.3390/antiox10060837

The influence of medical conditions like diabetes, cardiovascular disease, and obesity on the risk of ED

In our continuous journey towards understanding Erectile Dysfunction (ED), a condition that affects the ability to achieve or maintain an erection, it is critical to recognize the profound influence of certain medical conditions. Diabetes, cardiovascular disease, and obesity don't just impact general health, they can also significantly increase the risk of ED.[110,111]

Take diabetes as an example. This condition, especially when poorly managed, can lead to nerve damage and blood vessel deterioration, essential for achieving an erection. Similarly, cardiovascular diseases like coronary artery disease can obstruct blood flow to the penis, making it challenging to maintain an erection. It's not just these conditions, though - obesity plays a significant role, too. Excessive fat, particularly around the waist and in unusual places like the liver or pancreas, can disrupt hormone balance and blood circulation, thereby contributing to the development of ED.

Understanding the link between these medical conditions and ED is more than an academic endeavor. It's about

[110] Obesity and Erectile Dysfunction, NIH, Retrieved from: https://www.ncbi.nlm.nih.gov/pmc/articles/PMC6479091/
[111] Obesity and Cardiovascular Disease, Circulation, Retrieved from: https://www.ahajournals.org/doi/full/10.1161/CIR.0000000000000973

empowering you with knowledge to make informed decisions about your health. By managing these conditions effectively, you can significantly reduce your risk of ED. Remember, every step you take towards better health is a step away from ED. Your health, your power!

Psychological Contributors to ED

Erectile Dysfunction (ED) is not just a physical condition; it is also deeply intertwined with our emotional and psychological well-being. Factors such as stress, anxiety, depression, and relationship issues can significantly contribute to the development and persistence of ED.[112] Understanding these psychological triggers is vital in painting a complete picture of ED, empowering us to address the issue more effectively.

For instance, consider stress, which could be related to various aspects of life such as work, finances, or marital discord. Such stress can hinder a man's ability to achieve and maintain an erection. Similarly, anxiety can play a significant role in perpetuating ED. The fear of sexual failure and the resulting stress can create a vicious cycle that exacerbates ED. Depression is another crucial factor. It can both cause and

---

[112] Erectile Dysfunction, WebMd, Retrieved from: https://www.webmd.com/erectile-dysfunction/ed–psychological-causes

result from ED, impacting individuals on multiple fronts - physically and psychologically. Lastly, relationship issues, characterized by guilt, low self-esteem, or a loss of interest in sex, can also culminate in ED.[113]

Addressing these psychological factors is not merely about treating a symptom; it's about comprehensively managing a condition that affects millions of men worldwide. By integrating psychological treatment into the medical management of ED, we can help improve outcomes. This includes reducing anxiety, challenging negative beliefs, increasing sexual stimulation, and enhancing communication and relationship intimacy. Remember, every step taken toward understanding and managing these psychological contributors is a step toward reclaiming your sexual health. Your health, your power!

Risks Associated with Erectile Dysfunction

Physical health implications of ED

Erectile Dysfunction (ED), the persistent inability to achieve or maintain an erection firm enough for sexual intercourse, is a multifaceted condition with both physical and

---

[113] Sexual Medicine, NIH, Retrieved from:
https://www.ncbi.nlm.nih.gov/pmc/articles/PMC8766276/

psychological triggers. Physical causes include heart disease, high blood pressure, diabetes, obesity, and prescription medications. These conditions can hinder blood flow or nerve signals essential for an erection. Factors like tobacco use and alcoholism, sleep disorders, and treatments for prostate issues can further complicate the picture.[114] The interplay of these factors underscores the complexity of ED, reiterating the need for comprehensive medical evaluation and treatment.

An essential aspect of understanding ED is recognizing its potential as an early warning sign for cardiovascular disease. Conditions like heart disease and diabetes, along with lifestyle factors such as tobacco use and being overweight, can restrict blood flow to the veins and arteries. This can lead to both ED and cardiovascular problems.[115] Therefore, the onset of ED may serve as a wake-up call, indicating the presence of underlying health conditions that require immediate attention. Remember, early detection and intervention can significantly improve outcomes in cardiovascular disease. So, if you're experiencing ED, don't hesitate to seek medical help. Your health, your power!

---

[114] Erectile Dysfunction, Mayo Clinic.
[115] ipid.

Mental health impacts of ED

Erectile Dysfunction (ED) is not just a physical health issue but also a significant mental health concern. It can profoundly affect a man's self-perception and emotional well-being. Feelings of inadequacy and low self-esteem often emerge from the perceived inability to satisfy a partner sexually. This can negatively impact self-worth and trigger feelings of guilt, contributing to a cycle of distress that further exacerbates ED.[116]

Depression is another critical aspect linked to ED, significantly affecting a person's overall well-being due to the distress caused by the condition. Moreover, the strain ED places on relationships cannot be underestimated. Communication problems, decreased intimacy, and increased conflict between partners are common, leading to further emotional turmoil. These issues can create a vicious cycle of negative emotions and sexual performance anxiety, reinforcing the need for comprehensive ED management that integrates medical and psychological approaches.[117] Acknowledging these mental health impacts is the first step towards breaking the cycle and reclaiming your sexual health.

---

[116] Erectile Dysfunction, WebMd.
[117] A Psychosocial Approach to Erectile Dysfunction, NIH, Retrieved from:
https://www.ncbi.nlm.nih.gov/pmc/articles/PMC8766276/

Your health, your power!

It decreased sexual satisfaction as a result of ED.

Erectile Dysfunction (ED), a condition often shrouded in shame and silence, has far-reaching implications beyond the individual directly affected. One significant yet often overlooked consequence of ED is decreased sexual satisfaction, which impacts both the man experiencing ED and his partner. The onset of ED can lead to performance anxiety and fear of sexual failure, creating a self-perpetuating cycle that further exacerbates the condition. This reality can breed guilt and inadequacy and even result in a loss of interest in sex. What was once a source of intimacy and pleasure is becoming a source of stress and discord, significantly affecting the quality of life for the man with ED.

I want to bring light to an often-overlooked community as a veteran. A US study (1998) shows that veteran males aged 55-64 with ED had lower emotional, social, and physical functions "compared to aged-matched population norms, indicating a profound impairment in quality of life."[118] The study concluded that the veteran population is consistent with

---

[118] The Quality of Life and Economic Burden of Erectile Dysfunction, NIH, Retrieved from: https://www.ncbi.nlm.nih.gov/pmc/articles/PMC7901407

the clinical experience of poor physical health.[119]

The ripple effects of ED also extend to the partner, impacting their sexual satisfaction and overall relationship happiness. Studies have shown that female partners of men with ED often report lower levels of sexual desire, arousal, and orgasm, as well as decreased satisfaction in the sexual relationship. The decrease in sexual activity and ensuing relationship difficulties can further compound these adverse effects, leading to a significant decline in the couple's overall quality of life. Recognizing and addressing this aspect of ED is critical to developing comprehensive treatment plans that consider the emotional and relational dimensions of the condition alongside its physical manifestations. Your health, your power! Remember, seeking help is not a sign of weakness but of strength. You are not alone in this journey.

Impact of ED on Men Aged 50 and Over

Detailed explanation of ED in men over 50

Erectile Dysfunction (ED) is a prevalent condition that can significantly impact the lives of men aged 50 and over. Characterized by difficulty in achieving or maintaining an erection sufficient for satisfying sexual activity, ED can affect

---

[119] ipid.

men of all ages. However, the risk amplifies as men age, with over half of men between 40 and 70 experiencing some form of ED.[120] This condition can profoundly affect self-confidence, inducing stress and contributing to relationship problems.

The root causes of ED are multifaceted and can encompass physical and psychological factors. Physically, conditions like heart disease, high blood pressure, diabetes, obesity, and smoking can contribute to ED. On the psychological front, depression, anxiety, stress, and relationship problems can play a significant role. In many cases, ED results from a combination of both physical and psychological factors. For example, a man in his 50s may experience ED due to underlying heart disease (a physical factor), leading to anxiety about sexual performance (a psychological factor).

Diagnosing ED involves open discussions with a healthcare provider, a comprehensive physical examination, and thorough scrutiny of medical history. Treatment options include oral prescription medications, self-injections or urethral suppositories, vacuum penis pumps, and penile implants. Lifestyle modifications, such as managing chronic health conditions, quitting smoking, reducing stress, and seeking help for mental health concerns, can also be integral

---

[120] Erectile Dysfunction, Mayo Clinic.

to managing ED effectively.[121] Remember, your health, your power! Seeking help is not a sign of weakness but of strength. You are not alone in this journey.

Prevalence rates of ED in this demographic

The prevalence of Erectile Dysfunction (ED) in men over 50 is a significant concern, necessitating a deeper understanding and proactive measures. Real-world observational data from the United States reveal an unsettling trend: the prevalence of ED escalates with age, peaking within the 60-69 age group before gradually receding in older demographics. In a study examining medical claims data, a mere 5.6% of men aged 18 and above were diagnosed with ED or prescribed phosphodiesterase type 5 inhibitors (PDE5Is), a standard treatment for ED. However, this figure surges to 11.5% within the 60-69 age bracket, illustrating an increased propensity for ED in this demographic.[122]

It's crucial to note that men diagnosed with ED or undergoing treatment often exhibit a higher prevalence of comorbid conditions than those without ED. Hypertension,

---

[121] Erectile Dysfunction, NIDDKD, Retrieved from:
https://www.niddk.nih.gov/health-information/urologic-diseases/erectile-dysfunction
[122] Relationship Between Age and Erectile Dysfunction Diagnosis Or Treatment Using Real-World Observational Data In The United States, NIH, Retrieved from:
https://www.ncbi.nlm.nih.gov/pmc/articles/PMC5540144/

cardiovascular diseases, diabetes mellitus, depression, and benign prostatic hyperplasia are commonly observed in men with ED. This pattern implies that age-related comorbidities might play a significant role in the onset of ED in older men. Interestingly, age is an independent risk factor for ED diagnosis or treatment, even after accounting for comorbidities. Each additional decade of age significantly increases the odds of having an ED diagnosis or treatment, barring men aged 90 and above with lower odds. This underscores age's crucial role in developing ED in men over 50.[123]

These findings accentuate the need for healthcare providers to recognize the heightened prevalence of ED in older men and consider age-related comorbidities when assessing and treating ED. Early detection and management of ED can significantly enhance the quality of life for men in this demographic. Remember, your health, your power! Seeking help is not a sign of weakness but of strength. You are not alone in this journey.[124]

---

[123] ibid.
[124] ibid.

Quality of life considerations for men over 50 living with ED

Erectile Dysfunction (ED) is a medical condition characterized by the inability to achieve or maintain an erection sufficient for sexual intercourse. It's a prevalent issue that can affect men of all ages. Still, it is widespread in those aged 40 and above, individuals with diabetes, those with a high body mass index (BMI), individuals battling depression, the physically inactive, and smokers.[125]

Numerous factors can contribute to ED, including issues with the circulatory system, nervous system complications, endocrine system disorders, certain conditions or diseases, specific medications, and psychological or emotional conditions. The symptoms of ED can vary from difficulty in obtaining or keeping an erection, requiring substantial stimulation to maintain an erection, to a complete inability to get an erection.

Diagnosing ED typically involves a comprehensive review of your medical history, including medication use, history of depression or anxiety, stress levels, relationship problems, and the frequency and quality of erections. Additional tests

---

[125] Erectile Dysfunction, Cleveland Clinic, Retrieved from: https://my.clevelandclinic.org/health/diseases/10035-erectile-dysfunction

such as blood tests, penile Doppler ultrasound, penile biothesiometry, and other imaging tests may be conducted to confirm a diagnosis.[126]

Once diagnosed, treatment options are diverse and can range from lifestyle modifications like cardiovascular exercise, quitting smoking, and seeking help from a sex therapist to medical interventions such as oral medications, penile low-intensity focused shockwave therapy, injectable medications, vacuum constriction devices, testosterone replacement therapy, and penile implant procedures.

Lifestyle changes are often the first line of defense against ED. Reducing cholesterol, maintaining physical activity, securing a healthy weight, achieving high-quality sleep, eating healthy foods, stopping smoking, and reducing or stopping drinking can all significantly prevent and manage ED.[127]

The prognosis for ED is generally favorable, and it's important to remember that it is a treatable condition. However, it may not resolve independently and require lifestyle changes or treatment. If you're experiencing symptoms of ED, it's crucial to consult with a healthcare provider. In some cases, seeking emergency care may be

---

[126] ibid.
[127] ibid.

necessary.

It's also important to note that partner support and open communication can benefit individuals struggling with ED. And let's not forget about our veterans—a community often overlooked when discussing ED. They, too, need our understanding, support, and access to comprehensive treatment options.

Remember, your health, your power! Seeking help is not a sign of weakness but of strength. You are not alone on this journey. Let's work together to ensure all communities, including our veterans, receive the support they need to manage ED effectively.

Health risks for men over 50 with ED

Men aged 50 and over with erectile dysfunction (ED) are confronted with heightened health risks, mainly when dealing with comorbid conditions like diabetes, cardiovascular disease, and obesity. Research indicates that these conditions often coexist with ED and can exacerbate its adverse effects on overall health and well-being. For instance, diabetes is a frequent comorbidity in men with ED, leading to complications such as neuropathy and vascular dysfunction, which can further impair erectile function. It's been found that around 37% of men with type 2 diabetes experience ED, primarily due to the vascular and neuropathic complications associated with this condition (PMC, 2013).[128]

Cardiovascular disease, another prevalent comorbidity, is closely associated with ED. The underlying vascular issues contributing to heart disease can likewise affect erectile function, potentially as a precursor to more severe cardiovascular events. Obesity, often linked with both diabetes and cardiovascular disease, significantly contributes to the development and progression of ED. Excessive weight can induce hormonal imbalances, vascular problems, and reduced testosterone levels, all of which can contribute to erectile dysfunction. Furthermore, obesity is a significant risk factor for various health conditions, including cardiovascular disease and heart failure, and can lead to systolic dysfunction and heart failure with reduced ejection fraction (HFrEF). Obesity-related comorbidities like diabetes, sleep apnea, and hypoventilation syndrome can increase the risk for pulmonary hypertension and right ventricular and left ventricular failure.[129]

These findings underscore the importance of

---

[128] Erectile Dysfunction and Diabetes, NIH, Retrieved from: https://www.ncbi.nlm.nih.gov/pmc/articles/PMC3731873/
[129] Obesity and Cardiovascular Disease, Circulation.

comprehensive healthcare management for men over 50 with ED, especially those with comorbid conditions like diabetes, cardiovascular disease, and obesity. By effectively managing these conditions, healthcare providers can help mitigate their impact on ED and improve patients' quality of life. Remember, your health, your power! Seeking help is not a sign of weakness but of strength. You are not alone in this journey.

Managing Erectile Dysfunction

Medical interventions for managing ED.

Medical interventions are critical to managing Erectile Dysfunction (ED), particularly for men over 50. One of the most common types of medical treatments involves phosphodiesterase type 5 inhibitors, such as Viagra and Cialis. These medications increase blood flow to the penis, facilitating erections when a man is sexually stimulated. They are typically effective in 70% of men with ED, making them a popular first-line treatment option.[130]

Hormone therapy is another viable medical intervention, especially for men with low testosterone levels. Testosterone replacement therapy can help improve sexual interest and

---

[130] What Is Erectile Dysfunction?, Urology Care Foundation, Retrieved from: https://www.urologyhealth.org/urology-a-z/e/

induce erections. However, it's important to note that this treatment is only effective in men with low testosterone levels and should be administered under the supervision of a healthcare professional due to potential side effects.[131]

Penile injections, another treatment option, involve injecting medication directly into the side of the penis. This method induces an erection by widening the blood vessels, thereby increasing blood flow to the area. It's a highly effective treatment with up to 85% success rates. Despite its effectiveness, some men might find this method intimidating or uncomfortable, highlighting the importance of discussing all available options with a healthcare provider.[132]

These medical interventions, lifestyle modifications, and psychological support can significantly improve the quality of life for men living with ED. Remember, your health, your power! Seeking help is not a sign of weakness but of strength. You are not alone on this journey.

Surgical options for treating ED.

When medical interventions and lifestyle changes are not sufficient to manage Erectile Dysfunction (ED), surgical options can be considered. One such option is the use of penile

---

[131] ibid.
[132] ibid.

implants. These involve the placement of a rod, often made of silicone rubber, into the penis to facilitate an erection. There are two main types of penile implants: malleable implants and inflatable devices. Plastic implants provide a semi-erect state and are easy to use. In contrast, inflatable devices can create a fully erect state and offer discretion and ease of access. Penile implants have been shown to have high success rates and satisfaction levels among those undergoing ED treatment options.[133]

Vascular reconstruction surgery is another surgical treatment for ED, though it is less commonly performed. This procedure aims to restore blood flow to the penis by repairing damaged blood vessels. It is primarily recommended for young males with arterial damage due to injury or congenital abnormalities rather than those with ED caused by conditions like high blood pressure or diabetes. The long-term results of vascular reconstruction surgery vary, and it is considered a high-risk procedure (Springer, 2020).[134]

These surgical options, combined with medical interventions, lifestyle modifications, and psychological

---

[133] What Are the Treatment Options For Erectile Dysfunction?, Medical News Today, Retrieved from: https://www.medicalnewstoday.com/articles/323688

[134] Vascular (Arterial And Venous) Surgery For Erectile Dysfunction, Springer, Retrieved from: https://link.springer.com/chapter/10.1007/978-3-030-21447-0_50

support, can significantly improve the quality of life for men living with ED. Remember, your health, your power! Seeking help is not a sign of weakness but of strength. You are not alone on this journey.

Lifestyle interventions to treat and prevent ED.

Lifestyle interventions play a pivotal role in managing Erectile Dysfunction (ED), often augmenting the effectiveness of medical and surgical treatments. Regular exercise, for example, has been proven to enhance cardiovascular health, which is crucial for erectile function. A study conducted among veterans in addiction treatment found that regular exercise was associated with better physical health-related quality of life.[135] This finding is particularly relevant as it underscores the potential of physical activity in improving ED symptoms among veterans, a group that often grapples with unique health challenges.

Maintaining a healthy weight is another critical lifestyle intervention. Obesity is a known risk factor for ED, as it can lead to hormonal imbalances and vascular problems that impair erectile function. Quitting smoking and reducing

---

[135] Health-Related Quality Of Life Among Veterans In Addictions Treatment, NCBI, Retrieved from: https://www.ncbi.nlm.nih.gov/pmc/articles/PMC6725536/

alcohol consumption is also vital, as both habits can cause damage to the blood vessels, exacerbating ED. Moreover, stress management techniques such as mindfulness and cognitive-behavioral therapy can help alleviate psychological factors contributing to ED. When coupled with medical treatments, these interventions can significantly improve the quality of life and overall well-being of men living with ED, including those in the veteran community.

Remember, your health is your power! Taking steps toward healthier habits is not merely a sign of self-care but also an act of resilience. You are not alone in this journey. Together, we can navigate the path toward improved health and vitality.

Summary

Erectile Dysfunction (ED) is a condition that affects many men, including those in the veteran community. However, it can be effectively managed with the right combination of treatments and interventions. This includes medical interventions like phosphodiesterase type 5 inhibitors and hormone therapy, surgical options such as penile implants and vascular surgery, and lifestyle changes involving regular exercise, maintaining a healthy weight, quitting smoking, reducing alcohol consumption, and stress management. Remember, your health is your power! With the right tools and guidance, you can navigate this journey successfully.

Key Points Checklist for Chapter 5: Erectile Dysfunction

1. **Understand the Definition:** Familiarize yourself with Erectile Dysfunction (ED), a condition characterized by the inability to achieve or maintain an erection for satisfactory sexual performance.

2. **Identify Contributing Factors:** Explore the various factors contributing to ED, including genetic predispositions, environmental factors, medical conditions, and psychological contributors.

3. **Recognize the Risks:** Be aware of the risks associated with ED, such as physical health implications, mental health impacts, and decreased sexual satisfaction, and understand the importance of addressing these risks.

4. **Understand the Impact on Men aged 50 and Over:** Gain insights into how ED affects men aged 50 and over, including prevalence rates and detailed explanations of its impact on their lives.

5. **Explore Treatment Options:** Learn about different management approaches for ED, including medical interventions, surgical options, and lifestyle interventions, enabling you to make informed decisions regarding your health.

Call to Action:

Now that we've explored the vital ED information necessary for men over 50, it's time to implement this knowledge. Here's your five-step action plan:

1. **Seek Medical Help**: If you are experiencing symptoms of ED, contact a healthcare provider for

proper evaluation and diagnosis.

2. **Discuss Treatment Options:** Have an open conversation with your healthcare provider about available treatment options, including medications, hormone therapy, penile injections, penile implants, and vascular surgery, to find the best approach for your situation.

3. **Adopt Lifestyle Changes:** Take proactive steps towards managing ED by making lifestyle changes, such as engaging in regular exercise, maintaining a healthy weight, quitting smoking, reducing alcohol consumption, and effectively managing stress levels.

4. **Address Mental Health and Relationships:** Recognize the impact of ED on mental health and relationships and seek psychological support if needed. Remember, seeking help is a sign of strength and can greatly improve overall well-being.

5. **Remember You Are Not Alone:** Understand that ED is a treatable condition, and there are many others facing similar challenges. Reach out for support, connect with relevant communities, and remember that you can regain control of your sexual health and overall quality of life.

Chapter 6: Mental Health

"You are valuable just because you exist. Not because of what you do or have done, but simply because you are."

~ Max Lucado

In Micronesia, mental health issues among men have reached alarming levels, with the rate of psychotics per 10,000 adults standing at 54, a figure that is significantly higher than the global average.[136] Schizophrenia, the most common form of psychosis, accounts for 73% of these cases. The male-to-female ratio of psychosis in Micronesia is an astounding 3.4:1, underscoring the severity of mental health problems among men in this region.[137]

Table 1: Psychosis Rates by Island Group, 1980 and 1990

1978-1980	Palau	Yap	Chuuk	Pohnpei	Kosrae	Marsahalls	General
Pop (15 yrs +)	8,264	6,009	18,279	13,206	2,568	13,481	61,807
No. of Psychotics	78	50	44	25	4	12	213
Rate/10,000	94	83	24	19	16	9	34
1990							
Pop (15 yrs +)	7,666	6,289	24,490	17,476	4,061	21,244	81,224
No. of Psychotics	128	53	92	56	26	90	445
Rate/10,000	167	84	38	32	64	42	54

[Fig. 6-1: MicSem Publication]

---

[136] (1993) Mental Illness in Micronesia, MicSem Publications, Retrieved from: https://micsem.org/micronesian-counselo/mental-illness-in-micronesia/
[137] ibid.

Contrastingly, while men also face higher mental illness rates than women in the United States, the prevalence is somewhat lower. The suicide rate for males is 22.8 per 100,000 population, significantly less than the ratios observed in Micronesia.[138] Moreover, about 9.2% of adult men in the US have experienced a major depressive episode in the past year,[139] a figure that, while concerning, is somewhat less dire than the mental health crisis men face in Micronesia.

These statistics underscore the urgent need for targeted interventions and mental health support services tailored to address men's unique challenges in both regions. Despite the differences in magnitude and specific conditions, the common thread is clear: men's mental health is a critical issue that demands attention, understanding, and action.

Managing Stress and Anxiety with Healthy Habits

Exercise Regularly:

Regular exercise is considered one of the most efficient methods for managing stress and anxiety. Physical activity has numerous benefits for mental health, including reducing

---

[138] ibid.
[139] ibid.

stress hormones such as cortisol and adrenaline, increasing the release of endorphins, natural mood elevators, and improving sleep quality. Exercise enhances cognitive function, leading to better decision-making, problem-solving, and emotional regulation.[140]

Different types of exercise can benefit men over 50, including aerobic activities such as walking, swimming, and cycling, strength training, and flexibility exercises like yoga and Pilates. Choosing enjoyable and sustainable activities is essential to ensure long-term adherence to an exercise routine. To maintain a healthy lifestyle, the American Heart Association suggests moderate-intensity aerobic exercise for 150 minutes weekly or vigorous-intensity aerobic exercise for 75 minutes weekly, in addition to incorporating muscle-strengthening activities at least twice weekly. It is essential to seek guidance from a healthcare provider before commencing a new exercise routine, particularly for individuals with pre-existing medical conditions or physical constraints.

Practice Mindful Breathing and Relaxation Techniques:

Mindfulness practices, such as deep breathing and

---

[140] Biddle, S. J. H. (2016). Physical activity and mental health: evidence is growing. World Psychiatry, 15(2), 176–177. https://doi.org/10.1002/wps.20331

progressive muscle relaxation, are powerful tools for managing stress and anxiety. These techniques foster awareness and help individuals become more attuned to their thoughts, emotions, and bodily sensations. By focusing on the present moment and cultivating non-judgmental awareness, individuals can develop a more balanced perspective on their stressors and enhance their overall well-being.

Mindful breathing involves taking slow, deep breaths while focusing on the sensation of air entering and leaving the body. Activating the parasympathetic nervous system, which aids in promoting relaxation and minimizing the physiological manifestations of stress, can be facilitated through this approach. To practice mindful breathing, find a quiet and comfortable space and follow these steps:

- Assume a comfortable posture, either seated or lying down, and close your eyes or concentrate on a solitary point.
- Position one hand on your chest and the other on your abdomen.
- Inhale deeply and slowly through your nose, letting your abdomen expand as you fill your lungs with air.
- Exhale slowly through your mouth or nose, feeling your abdomen fall as you release breath.
- Practice this exercise for a few minutes, concentrating on the feeling of your breath as it flows in and out of your body.

Progressive muscle relaxation is an additional technique involving the tensing and subsequent release of various muscle groups to ease tension and encourage relaxation. This technique can be beneficial for individuals who retain stress-related body tension.

To practice progressive muscle relaxation, follow these steps:

- Find a quiet, comfortable space to sit or lie down.
- Begin by focusing on your breath, taking slow, deep breaths in and out.
- Begin at your feet and progress upward through your body, tensing and then relaxing each group of muscles sequentially.
- As you tense each muscle, hold the tension for about 5 seconds, and then release the pressure as you exhale, feeling the muscles relax.
- Continue this process for each muscle group, up to your head and face.

Integrating these relaxation methods into your everyday routine can greatly influence stress and anxiety levels, supporting men over 50 in preserving good mental health and overall wellness.[141]

---

[141] Goyal, M., Singh, S., Sibinga, E. M., Gould, N. F., Rowland-Seymour, A., Sharma, R., ... & Haythornthwaite, J. A. (2014). Meditation programs for psychological stress and well-being: a systematic review and meta-analysis. JAMA Internal Medicine, 174(3), 357–368. https://doi.org/10.1001/jamainternmed.2013.13018

Talk to a Therapist:

Obtaining professional assistance from a therapist or counselor can be highly advantageous in managing stress and anxiety. Therapists can provide guidance and support in identifying the sources of stress, developing effective coping strategies, and improving emotional well-being. Cognitive-behavioral therapy (CBT) successfully treats anxiety disorders and stress-related concerns.[142]

Through CBT, individuals learn to identify and challenge negative thought patterns, develop problem-solving skills, and practice relaxation techniques. For men over 50, working with a therapist can provide invaluable tools to navigate the challenges of aging and maintain good mental health.

Get Adequate Sleep:

Sleep is a priority for maintaining good mental health and managing stress. Insufficient sleep can intensify stress and anxiety; however, sufficient sleep supports emotional regulation and cognitive functioning. Strive for 7-9 hours of sleep per night, as the National Sleep Foundation advises. Creating a regular bedtime routine can enhance sleep quality and alleviate stress. Establishing a consistent bedtime routine

---

[142] Hofmann, S. G., Asnaani, A., Vonk, I. J., Sawyer, A. T., & Fang, A. (2012). The efficacy of cognitive behavioral therapy: A review of meta-analyses. *Cognitive therapy and research*, 36, 427-440.

can help improve sleep quality and reduce stress. This routine may include relaxation practices, such as deep breathing exercises or progressive muscle relaxation, creating a comfortable sleep environment free of distractions, and avoiding stimulants like caffeine and nicotine close to bedtime.

To maintain good sleep hygiene, it is crucial to adhere to a consistent sleep schedule by sleeping and waking up at the same time every day, even on weekends. This practice can aid in regulating the body's internal clock, thus facilitating ease in falling asleep and feeling refreshed. In cases of persistent difficulties with sleep, it is recommended to seek medical advice to diagnose any underlying problems and develop a plan for enhancing sleep quality.

Practice Healthy Eating Habits:

A well-balanced diet can significantly impact mental health and stress management. Eating various nutrient-dense foods, such as fruits, vegetables, healthy fats, lean proteins, and whole grains, can supply the vital nutrients required for optimal brain function and emotional well-being. Studies indicate that a diet high in fruits, vegetables, whole grains, and lean proteins is linked with a reduced risk of depression and anxiety.[143] In addition to following a well-balanced diet, it is crucial to practice portion control and avoid emotional eating, which can be triggered by stress. Emotional eating can lead to weight gain and further exacerbate stress levels. Instead, prioritize mindful eating habits, such as eating slowly, relishing every bite, and being attentive to hunger and fullness signals. This approach can encourage a healthier relationship with food and facilitate better mental health.

Incorporating these healthy habits into your everyday routine can assist in managing stress and anxiety, improving mental health and overall well-being for men over 50. By prioritizing self-care, seeking professional help, and adopting effective coping strategies, men can maintain good mental health as they age.

Schedule Time for Yourself Each Day:

It is essential to allocate time for self-care and relaxation to maintain mental health and manage stress. Scheduling regular *me time* allows individuals to engage in activities that bring joy, promote peace, and recharge their mental and emotional batteries. Men over 50 must prioritize their well-

---

[143] Lassale, C., Batty, G. D., Baghdadli, A., Jacka, F., Sánchez-Villegas, A., Kivimäki, M., & Akbaraly, T. (2019). Healthy dietary indices and risk of depressive outcomes: a systematic review and meta-analysis of observational studies. Molecular Psychiatry, 24(7), 965-986. https://doi.org/10.1038/s41380-018-0237-8

being and ensure they have time for themselves amidst their daily responsibilities.

Setting aside even 15 to 30 minutes per day for self-care can make a significant difference in managing stress levels. Activities during this time may include reading, journaling, taking a leisurely walk, or simply enjoying a cup of coffee or tea in solitude. These moments of self-care can help cultivate a sense of inner peace and balance, ultimately promoting better mental health and well-being.

Find an Outlet or Hobby to Relax and Destress:

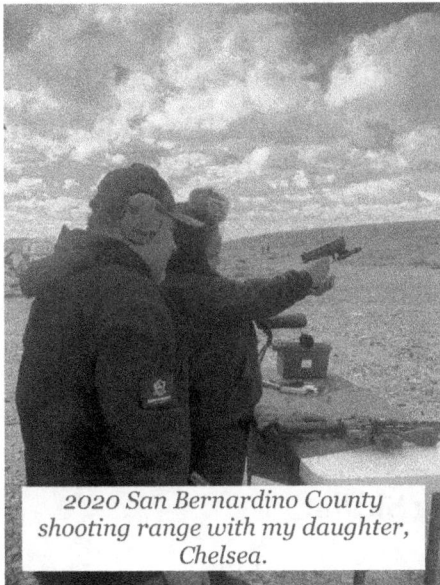
2020 San Bernardino County shooting range with my daughter, Chelsea.

Engaging in hobbies and leisure activities can be a powerful way to relieve stress and maintain mental health. Hobbies provide a sense of accomplishment, foster creativity, and help individuals feel more in control of their lives. For men over 50, participating in enjoyable activities can provide a much-needed break from everyday stressors and promote a sense of purpose and fulfillment.

Various hobbies and activities include gardening, painting, playing a musical instrument, woodworking, and cooking. The crucial aspect is discovering an enjoyable activity that enables individuals to be present and disregard their stressors. Research has shown that participating in leisure activities can reduce stress levels, decrease the risk of depression, and improve overall mental health.[144] In conclusion, adopting healthy habits, such as exercising regularly, practicing mindful breathing, talking to a therapist, getting adequate sleep, and eating well, can significantly improve mental health and reduce stress for men over 50. Additionally, scheduling time for self-care and engaging in enjoyable hobbies can provide a much-needed respite from daily stressors and promote overall well-being. By prioritizing mental health and implementing these strategies, men over 50 can navigate the challenges of aging with resilience and maintain a positive outlook on life.

Developing Positive Coping Mechanisms & Strategies

Develop Problem-Solving Skills:

Cultivating practical problem-solving skills can enhance

---

[144] American Psychological Association. (2021). Stress Management. Retrieved from: https://www.apa.org/topics/stress

one's resilience and improve one's ability to cope with life's challenges, especially for men over 50 who may face unique stressors related to aging, such as changes in physical health, social roles, and personal relationships. Problem-solving involves identifying problems, generating possible solutions, evaluating the potential outcomes of each solution, and implementing the chosen solution. By developing these skills, individuals can feel more in control of their lives and be better equipped to manage stress and anxiety. One approach to improving problem-solving skills is to adopt a structured method, which includes the following steps:

- Define the problem: Identify your issue or challenge.

- Generate possible solutions: Brainstorm multiple solutions to the problem without judgment, considering various perspectives and approaches.

- Evaluate the solutions: Weigh the pros and cons of each potential solution, considering the possible outcomes and consequences.

- Choose the best solution: Given the circumstances, select the most appropriate and feasible solution.

- Implement the solution: Take action to put the chosen solution into practice, monitoring the results and adjusting as necessary.

- Reflect on the process: Assess the effectiveness of the chosen solution and learn from the experience to improve future problem-solving efforts.

Identify and Challenge Negative Thoughts:

Negative thinking patterns, often called cognitive distortions, can contribute to stress and anxiety. These patterns include all-or-nothing thinking, catastrophizing, and personalization, among others. Individuals can develop a more balanced and realistic perspective by learning to identify and challenge these thought patterns, ultimately reducing stress and improving mental health. Cognitive-behavioral therapy (CBT) techniques can help identify and challenge negative thoughts. One effective technique is the "ABCDE" model, which involves the following steps:

- Identify the activating event or situation that triggered the negative thought.

- Recognize the belief or negative thought associated with the event.

- Observe the consequences or emotional reactions resulting from the belief.

- Dispute or challenge negative thoughts by considering alternative explanations, evidence, or perspectives.

- Establish a new, more balanced thought or belief based on the alternative information.[145]

Practice Positive Self-Talk:

Positive self-talk is a powerful tool for managing stress and anxiety and promoting better mental health. Individuals can cultivate a healthier mindset and improve their well-being by consciously shifting their internal dialogue toward more positive and supportive messages. For men over 50, positive self-talk can be particularly beneficial for navigating the challenges of aging and maintaining a positive outlook on life.

To practice positive self-talk, consider the following strategies:

- Replace negative self-statements with positive or neutral ones: Instead of saying, "I can't do this," try saying, "This is challenging, but I can work through it."

- Focus on your strengths and accomplishments: Remind yourself of your successes and the qualities that make you unique and capable.

- Use affirmations: Repeat positive statements to yourself, such as "I am capable," "I am worthy," or "I

[145] Hofmann, S. G., Asnaani, A., Vonk, I. J., Sawyer, A. T., & Fang, A. (2012). The efficacy of cognitive–behavioral therapy: A review of meta–analyses.

can handle this situation."

- Challenge irrational beliefs: When you notice negative thoughts, question their validity and consider alternative explanations.

- Nurture self-compassion: Treat yourself with kindness and empathy. Acknowledge that everyone confronts obstacles and makes mistakes.

By implementing these strategies, men over 50 can develop positive coping mechanisms and techniques to effectively manage stress and anxiety, promoting better mental health and overall well-being.

Engage in Activities that Promote Positive Emotions:

Participating in activities that foster positive emotions can significantly improve mental health and well-being, especially for men over 50 who may face unique challenges associated with aging. Fostering positive emotions, such as joy, gratitude, and contentment, can counterbalance the adverse impacts of stress and anxiety, ultimately enhancing resilience and emotional equilibrium. Furthermore, positive emotions have been linked to numerous psychological and physical health benefits, including improved immune function, reduced inflammation, and increased longevity.[146]

Some activities that can promote positive emotions include:

- Expressing gratitude: Keep a gratitude journal or share your appreciation with others regularly. Focusing on the positive aspects of life can help cultivate a more optimistic outlook.

- Engaging in acts of kindness: Doing big and small acts can boost positive emotions and foster a sense of connectedness with others.

- Practicing mindfulness: Mindfulness meditation or mindful activities, such as yoga, can help individuals fully experience positive emotions by promoting a nonjudgmental awareness of the present moment.

- Nurturing social connections: Investing time and effort in building strong relationships with friends and family can provide a vital source of support, happiness, and positive emotions.

---

[146] Kok, B. E., Coffey, K. A., Cohn, M. A., Catalino, L. I., Vacharkulksemsuk, T., Algoe, S. B., ... & Fredrickson, B. L. (2013). How positive emotions build physical health: Perceived positive social connections account for the upward spiral between positive emotions and vagal tone. Psychological Science, 24(7), 1123–1132. https://doi.org/10.1177/0956797612470827

- Pursuing hobbies and interests: Enjoyable and personally meaningful activities can promote a sense of accomplishment, pleasure, and positive emotions.

Learn How to Set Boundaries and Limits:

Healthy boundaries are essential for maintaining mental health and managing stress, particularly for men over 50 who may face numerous demands and responsibilities.

Boundaries help individuals establish a sense of balance, protect their emotional well-being, and maintain positive relationships with others.

To set effective boundaries and limits, consider the following tips:

- Identify your values and priorities: Determine what is most important to you in various aspects of your life, such as work, family, and personal growth. This can help you make decisions about where to set boundaries.

- Communicate your needs: Clearly express your needs and preferences to others, using assertive communication techniques that convey your message without being aggressive or passive.

- Be consistent and firm: Uphold your boundaries by reinforcing them, even when difficult or uncomfortable.

This may involve saying "no" to requests or declining invitations infringing on your time or well-being.

- Practice self-compassion: Recognize that setting boundaries is essential to self-care and self-respect. Give yourself permission to prioritize your well-being and understand that it is not selfish to do so.

- Seek support: Discuss your boundaries and limits with trusted friends, family members, or a mental health professional who can provide encouragement and guidance.

By engaging in activities promoting positive emotions and learning to set healthy boundaries, men over 50 can develop effective coping strategies to manage stress and anxiety, ultimately improving their mental health and well-being.

Find Ways to Practice Self-Compassion:

Practicing self-compassion is vital for sustaining good mental health and dealing with stress and anxiety, particularly for men over 50 who may encounter distinctive challenges related to aging. Self-compassion encompasses treating oneself with kindness, empathy, and a lack of judgment, especially during trying times. Studies indicate that self-compassion is linked to lower symptoms of anxiety and depression, greater resilience, and enhanced overall well-being.[147]

To cultivate self-compassion, consider the following strategies:

- Mindfulness: Develop an awareness of your thoughts and feelings without judgment, recognizing that they are natural and universal experiences. This can help create space for self-compassion to emerge.

- Self-kindness: Treat yourself with the same kindness and understanding that you would offer a close friend or loved one who is struggling. Acknowledge your feelings without harsh criticism or self-blame.

- Common humanity: Remember that everyone experiences difficulties, setbacks, and imperfections. Recognize that your struggles are a part of the shared human experience, fostering a sense of connection and empathy.

Find Support from Friends and Family:

Establishing a robust support network of friends and family is crucial for sustaining mental health and managing stress and anxiety. Social support can offer emotional

---

[147] Neff, K. D., & Germer, C. K. (2013). A pilot study and randomized controlled trial of the mindful self-compassion program. Journal of Clinical Psychology, 69(1), 28–44. https://doi.org/10.1002/jclp.21923

encouragement, practical aid, and a feeling of belonging, all contributing to enhanced mental health and well-being. For men over 50, having a solid support network can be particularly beneficial in navigating the challenges of aging and maintaining a positive outlook on life. To strengthen connections with friends and family and build a support network, consider the following tips:

- Be proactive in nurturing relationships: Reach out to friends and family members regularly to maintain connections, share experiences, and offer support.

- Develop new connections: Join clubs, organizations, or community groups that interest you to meet new people and expand your social circle.

- Be open and vulnerable: Share your feelings, challenges, and concerns with trusted friends and family members, allowing them to provide support and understanding.

- Offer support to others: Be available to listen, empathize, and provide encouragement to friends and family members who are facing their challenges. Offering help can deepen relationships and foster a sense of reciprocity.

- Seek professional help when needed: If you are struggling to cope with stress and anxiety, consider contacting a mental health professional who can provide guidance, support, and effective coping strategies.

By practicing self-compassion and building a solid support network of friends and family, men over 50 can develop effective coping mechanisms to manage stress and anxiety, ultimately promoting better mental health and overall well-being.

Practicing Self-Care & Self-Compassion:

Set Realistic Goals for Yourself:

Establishing realistic and achievable goals is an essential aspect of self-care and self-compassion, particularly for men over 50 who may face unique challenges related to aging. By setting manageable goals, individuals can maintain motivation, foster a sense of accomplishment, and reduce the risk of becoming overwhelmed or discouraged. Furthermore, pursuing goals aligning with one's values and priorities can promote personal growth and well-being.

To set realistic goals, consider the following strategies:

- Divide significant objectives into smaller, more

achievable tasks: Concentrating on smaller tasks can help you progress toward your larger goal without feeling overwhelmed.

- Use the SMART criteria: Make your goals Specific, Measurable, Achievable, Relevant, and Time-bound. This can help ensure that your goals are well-defined and attainable.

- Adjust your goals as needed: Be flexible and willing to revise your goals if circumstances change or you encounter unforeseen obstacles. This can help maintain motivation and prevent feelings of failure or frustration.

- Celebrate your accomplishments: Acknowledge and reward yourself for achieving your goals, even the small ones. This can help reinforce your efforts and maintain motivation.

Take Time to Rest and Relax:

Prioritizing relaxation is crucial for maintaining mental health and managing stress, especially for men over 50, who may face aging-related stressors. Rest can help individuals recharge, gain perspective, and reduce chronic stress's harmful effects on physical and mental health.

To ensure that you take adequate time to rest and relax, consider implementing the following strategies:

- Schedule regular breaks: Set aside designated times for relaxation and self-care activities throughout the day or week. Treat these times as non-negotiable appointments with yourself.

- Develop a relaxation routine: Create a routine that incorporates relaxation techniques or activities that you enjoy, such as reading, taking a bath, meditating, or going for a leisurely walk.

- Practice good sleep hygiene: Establish a consistent sleep schedule, create a comfortable sleep environment, and develop a relaxing bedtime routine to promote better sleep quality.

- Listen to your body: Pay attention to your body's signals for rest, such as fatigue or tension, and prioritize self-care accordingly.

Engage in activities that promote relaxation: Consider trying activities such as yoga, tai chi, or mindfulness meditation, which have been shown to reduce stress and promote peace.[148] By setting realistic goals and prioritizing rest, men over 50 can practice self-care and self-compassion, effectively managing stress and promoting better mental health and overall well-being.

Incorporate Enjoyable Activities into your Schedule:

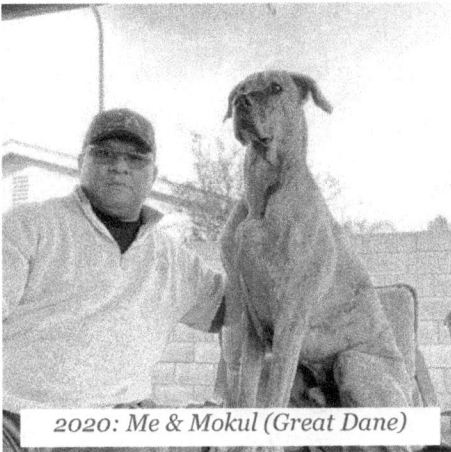

2020: Me & Mokul (Great Dane)

Engaging in enjoyable activities is a vital component of self-care and self-compassion, particularly for men over 50 who may experience increased stress and challenges related to aging. Enjoyable activities can provide a much-needed respite from stress, boost mood, and promote overall well-being. You can balance work, responsibilities, and leisure by incorporating enjoyable activities into your daily or weekly schedule. Some tips for incorporating enjoyable activities into your plan include:

---

[148] Pascoe, M. C., & Bauer, I. E. (2015). A systematic review of randomised control trials on the effects of yoga on stress measures and mood. Journal of Psychiatric Research, 68, 270–282. https://doi.org/10.1016/j.jpsychires.2015.07.013

- Prioritize activities that align with your interests and values: Choose activities that genuinely bring you joy, satisfaction, and a sense of accomplishment.

- Set aside dedicated time for leisure: Schedule regular blocks for enjoyable activities, treating them as essential and non-negotiable commitments.

- Explore new interests and hobbies: Explore new activities that pique your curiosity, as they can provide fresh sources of enjoyment and personal growth.

- Invite friends and family to join you: Sharing enjoyable activities with loved ones can help strengthen social connections and enhance the overall experience.

Develop a Positive Body Image:

A positive body image is crucial for overall mental health and self-compassion, especially for men over 50 who may encounter age-related alterations in their physical appearance and capabilities. Cultivating a positive body image involves focusing on your body's functionality, strength, and resilience rather than solely on its appearance.[149]

To develop a positive body image, consider the following

---

[149] Frost, J., & McKelvie, S. (2014). Self-esteem and body satisfaction in male and female elementary school, high school, and university students. Sex Roles, 71(1-2), 45-54. https://doi.org/10.1007/s11199-014-0341-3

strategies:

- Practice gratitude for your body: Acknowledge and appreciate how your body supports you daily, from essential functions like breathing to more complex tasks like physical activities.

- Focus on what your body can do: Shift your attention from appearance to the abilities and strengths of your body, celebrating its accomplishments and resilience.

- Engage in physical activities that you enjoy: Participate in exercise or sports that bring you joy and help you feel strong, capable, and confident in your body.

- Challenge societal beauty standards: Recognize that media representations of physical beauty are often unrealistic and unattainable. Focus instead on cultivating your own unique sense of self-worth and attractiveness.

Seek Professional Help When Needed:

Recognizing when professional help is needed and seeking support from mental health professionals is essential to self-care and self-compassion. Men over 50 may encounter unique stressors and challenges related to aging, and accessing professional help can provide valuable guidance, coping strategies, and support to navigate these difficulties.

Consider seeking professional help if you experience any of the following:

- Persistent sadness, anxiety, or stress interfere with daily functioning.

- Difficulty coping with life transitions, such as retirement or losing a loved one.

- Struggles with body image or disordered eating behaviors.

- Relationship difficulties or concerns about social isolation.

- Any other mental health concerns that negatively impact your well-being.

By incorporating enjoyable activities into their schedule, developing a positive body image, and seeking professional help, men over 50 can practice self-care and self-compassion, effectively manage stress, and attain better mental health and overall well-being.

Make Time for Yourself Each Day to do Something that Brings You Joy:

Allocating time daily for activities that bring joy and fulfillment is critical for self-care and self-compassion, especially for men over 50 who may encounter heightened stress and challenges related to aging.

Engaging in activities that bring joy can help counterbalance the adverse effects of stress, improve mood, and enhance overall well-being.

To ensure that you make time for yourself each day, consider the following tips:

- Schedule daily *me time*: Treat time for yourself as an essential appointment in your daily routine. This can help ensure you prioritize your well-being amidst competing demands and responsibilities.

- Choose activities that align with your values and interests: Engage in activities that genuinely bring you happiness and satisfaction, whether reading a book, listening to music, gardening, or pursuing a creative hobby.

- Set boundaries with work and other obligations: Establish limits on your availability for work and other commitments, allowing yourself the necessary time and space to recharge and engage in enjoyable activities.

Prioritize your Health and Well-Being:

Focusing on overall health and well-being is essential to

self-care and self-compassion, especially for men over 50 who may face unique health challenges related to aging. Prioritizing your health involves taking proactive steps to maintain both physical and mental well-being, ultimately contributing to a better quality of life.

To prioritize your health and well-being, consider the following strategies:

- Adopt a balanced diet: Focus on consuming various nutrient-rich foods, including fruits, vegetables, whole grains, lean proteins, and healthy fats, to support overall health and well-being.[150]

- Incorporating consistent physical activity into your routine is crucial: The recommended amount of exercise includes 150 minutes of moderate-intensity aerobic activity per week or 75 minutes of vigorous-intensity aerobic activity per week and muscle-strengthening activities on two or more days per week.

- Maintain regular check-ups and screenings: Visit your healthcare provider regularly for check-ups,

---

[150] National Institute on Aging. (2020). Tips to boost your health as you age. U.S. Department of Health and Human Services. Retrieved from https://www.nia.nih.gov/health/infographics/tips-boost-your-health-you-age

vaccinations, and age-appropriate screenings to prevent and manage potential health issues.

- Address mental health concerns: Seek support from mental health professionals if you experience persistent stress, anxiety, or depression or encounter difficulties coping with life transitions or other challenges.

By making time for yourself each day to do something that brings you joy and prioritizing your health and well-being, men over 50 can practice self-care and self-compassion, effectively managing stress and promoting better mental health and overall well-being.

Key Points Checklist for Chapter 6: Mental Health

1. **Regular Exercise**: Prioritize physical activity, including aerobic exercises, strength training, and flexibility workouts. Regular exercise can significantly contribute to maintaining mental wellness by reducing anxiety, depression, and negative moods.

2. **Mindful Breathing and Relaxation Techniques**: Embrace deep breathing and progressive muscle relaxation techniques. These practices can help manage stress levels, promote relaxation, and improve mental health.

3. **Professional Guidance**: Don't hesitate to seek professional help from therapists or counselors. Their guidance and support can be instrumental in navigating mental health challenges.

4. **Adequate Sleep**: Ensure you get enough sleep by establishing a consistent sleep schedule and a relaxing bedtime routine. Quality sleep is crucial for mental well-being.

5. **Healthy Eating Habits**: Maintain a balanced diet and practice portion control. Proper nutrition plays a crucial role in supporting good mental health.

Call to Action:

Now that we've delved into the essential components of maintaining mental health, it's time to implement this knowledge. Here's your five-step action plan:

1. **Self-Care is Non-Negotiable**: Prioritize self-care and avoid seeking professional help when needed.

Mental health matters, and caring for your mind is just as important as caring for your body.

2. **Incorporate Joyful Activities**: Include activities that bring you joy in your daily routine. Engaging in enjoyable experiences can boost your mood and foster positive mental health.

3. **Celebrate Your Achievements**: Set realistic goals, and don't forget to acknowledge your accomplishments, no matter how small. Every step forward is a milestone in your mental health journey.

4. **Take Time for Yourself**: Dedicate daily to do something that brings you peace and happiness. Remember, your time is valuable, and so are you.

5. **Prioritize Your Overall Health**: Embrace a balanced diet, engage in regular physical activity, and promptly address mental health concerns. Your well-being is the cornerstone of a fulfilling life.

In the journey to mental wellness, every step you take matters. Implement this checklist and make your mental health a priority. Remember, maintaining mental health is not a destination but a continuous journey of self-care, understanding, and resilience. Let's commit to this journey together because your mental health matters!

Chapter 7: Social Health

"You can make more friends in two months by becoming interested in other people than you can in two years by trying to get others interested in you."

~Dale Carnegie

The Importance of Social Engagement for Men Over 50

As men enter their fifties, life can change physically and emotionally. The importance of staying socially engaged must be addressed during this time. Social engagement plays a crucial role in maintaining mental health and overall well-being. Men over 50 who engage in social activities with friends, family, or community members are more likely to lead happier, healthier, and more fulfilling lives.

Research has shown that social engagement can significantly impact various aspects of health, particularly for older adults. Engaging in frequent social interactions can aid in maintaining mental acuity and improving cognitive abilities, which may lead to a decreased likelihood of experiencing cognitive impairment and the onset of dementia. It can also help to alleviate feelings of loneliness, depression, and anxiety—all of which can negatively impact overall health and quality of life.

Reflecting on my life, I recall the momentous decision over 30 years ago when I left the comforting embrace of Kosrae, my tiny island home in Micronesia, to venture into new horizons in the United States. The journey was filled with promise and anticipation but also meant leaving behind a cherished lifestyle that held family and community at its heart.

In my homeland, we revered our elders, caring for them

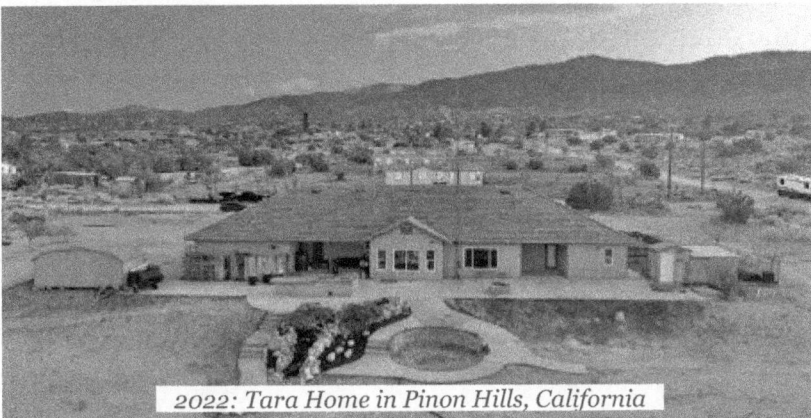

2022: Tara Home in Pinon Hills, California

within our homes as an integral part of our extended family fabric. It was a practice rooted in love, respect, and a deep sense of duty. However, the landscape of elder care is starkly different in the U.S., where nursing homes are more common. This shift was difficult for me to reconcile with, as I yearned for the close-knit familial bonds of my upbringing.

I decided to bridge this cultural chasm in my way. Inspired

by the values of my homeland and driven by a deep personal conviction, I invited my 81-year-old mother to live with us in our seven-bedroom home on a four-acre piece of land in Southern California. In doing so, I sought to recreate a slice of Kosrae in the heart of California, upholding our tradition of caring for our elders within the family fold. This decision has brought immense joy and warmth to our home and allowed me to impart the invaluable lessons of respect and care for older adults to my four children. Through this journey, I have strived to blend the best of both worlds, cherishing my roots while adapting to my adopted home.

The Benefits of Staying Socially Connected

There are numerous benefits to staying socially connected, particularly for men over 50. Some of these benefits include:

1. Improved mental health: Consistent social engagements can enhance one's emotional well-being and counteract isolation, despondency, and apprehension.

2. Enhanced cognitive function: Sustaining social involvement may preserve cognitive performance and potentially lower the chances of developing cognitive deterioration and dementia.

3. Stronger immune system: Research has associated

social connections with a reinforced immune system, assisting men aged 50 and above in sustaining optimal overall health.[151]

4. Increased longevity: Individuals who cultivate robust social networks typically enjoy longer and healthier lives compared to those who experience more excellent social seclusion.[152]

5. Better physical health: Social engagement can lead to increased physical activity, which promotes better overall health and can help to prevent or manage chronic health conditions.

In the subsequent sections, we will explore different tactics to establish connections with others and construct a dependable support system of friends and family, enabling men aged 50 and above to sustain a dynamic and wholesome way of living.

Connecting with Others at Any Age:

Reach Out to Family and Friends:

---

[151] Cohen, S., Doyle, W. J., Skoner, D. P., Rabin, B. S., & Gwaltney, J. M., Jr (1997). Social ties and susceptibility to the common cold. JAMA, 277(24), 1940-1944. https://doi.org/10.1001/jama.1997.03540480040036

[152] Holt-Lunstad, J., Smith, T. B., & Layton, J. B. (2010). Social relationships and mortality risk: A meta-analytic review. PLoS Medicine, 7(7), e1000316. https://doi.org/10.1371/journal.pmed.1000316

Schedule regular phone calls or visits.

One of the easiest ways to stay socially engaged is to maintain regular contact with family and friends. Schedule weekly or monthly phone calls, video chats, or face-to-face visits with loved ones. Establishing a schedule can increase the probability of adhering to these social engagements, furnishing you with regular opportunities for social interaction.[153]

Attend family gatherings and events.

Family gatherings, such as birthdays, holidays, and reunions, provide excellent opportunities for socializing and connecting with loved ones. Make an effort to attend these events whenever possible, even if it requires extra planning or travel. Participating in family events can help strengthen bonds and create lasting memories.

Join a Club or Organization:

Find groups with shared interests.

Exploring hobbies and interests can facilitate the formation of fresh social connections. You can seek out nearby clubs or organizations that correspond to your interests, such as gardening clubs, photography groups, or book clubs.

---

[153] National Institute on Aging. (2021). Staying connected. U.S. Department of Health and Human Services. https://www.nia.nih.gov/health/staying-connected

Engaging in activities that bring you joy alongside individuals who share your interests can foster a sense of affiliation and furnish significant social interaction.

Attend meetings and events.

Once you have found a club or organization that aligns with your interests, make an effort to attend meetings and events regularly. This not only helps to maintain social connections but can also provide opportunities for personal growth and development. Research suggests that staying socially engaged during later stages of life can enhance cognitive function and contribute to overall well-being.[154] Attending meetings and events lets you stay connected, learn new skills, and expand your social circle. Connecting with others is essential for men over 50. By reaching out to family and friends, joining clubs or organizations, and attending meetings and events, you can maintain an active social life and enjoy the numerous benefits of social engagement.

Volunteer in the Community:

---

[154] Holt-Lunstad, J. (2017). The potential public health relevance of social isolation and loneliness: Prevalence, epidemiology, and risk factors. Public Policy & Aging Report, 27(4), 127-130. https://doi.org/10.1093/ppar/prx030

Find local organizations and causes.

Volunteering is an excellent way to stay socially engaged while positively impacting your community. Research local organizations and causes that resonate with your values and interests. Nonprofit organizations, community centers, hospitals, and schools often rely on volunteers for various tasks and programs. Websites such as VolunteerMatch.org can help connect you with opportunities in your area. Volunteering allows you to meet new people, engage in meaningful work, and establish a sense of purpose in your life.

Give back and make a difference.

Contributing to your community through volunteering can provide a profound sense of fulfillment and accomplishment. Studies have shown that volunteer individuals experience higher levels of life satisfaction, self-esteem, and overall well-being.[155] By volunteering and contributing to your community, you can make a concrete impact on the lives of others while nurturing your own personal development.

---

[155] Thoits, P. A., & Hewitt, L. N. (2001). Volunteer work and well-being. Journal of Health and Social Behavior, 42(2), 115-131. https://doi.org/10.2307/3090173

Try Something New, Such as a Hobby, Class, or Activity:

Explore new interests.

One way to stay socially engaged and maintain cognitive health is to explore new interests and activities continually. Trying something new can be exciting and invigorating, whether taking up a new hobby, learning a new skill, or participating in a new physical activity. Not only can this help to expand your social circle, but it can also keep your mind sharp and challenged.[156]

Learn new skills and meet new people.

Taking classes or participating in workshops can provide opportunities to learn new skills and connect with others who share your interests. Local community centers, colleges, or specialized schools often offer various art, music, cooking, or dance courses. Additionally, lifelong learning programs for older adults can provide various educational and enrichment opportunities. Pursuing new skills and interests allows you to meet new people, develop lasting friendships, and maintain an active, socially engaged lifestyle.

---

[156] Park, D. C., Lodi–Smith, J., Drew, L., Haber, S., Hebrank, A., Bischof, G. N., & Aamodt, W. (2014). The impact of sustained engagement on cognitive function in older adults: The Synapse Project. Psychological Science, 25(1), 103–112. https://doi.org/10.1177/0956797613499592

Staying socially engaged as a man over 50 is vital for overall health and well-being. Volunteering in the community and trying new hobbies, classes, or activities can help you build and maintain a robust social network. Embrace the opportunities to give back, explore new interests, and connect with others as you navigate this stage of life.

Take Advantage of Technology to Connect Remotely:

Utilize video chats, social media, and online forums.

In the current era of digitalization, technology has simplified the process of maintaining contact with friends, family, and groups of shared interests, even in situations where physical proximity is not feasible. Video chat platforms like Zoom, Skype, or FaceTime enable face-to-face conversations, helping maintain relationships and providing a sense of presence.[157] Engaging in video chats can help alleviate loneliness and improve overall well-being.

You can leverage social media platforms such as Facebook, Twitter, and Instagram to maintain connections with friends

---

[157] Nowland, R., Necka, E. A., & Cacioppo, J. T. (2018). Loneliness and social internet use: Pathways to reconnection in a digital world? erspectives on Psychological Science, 13(1), 70–87. https://doi.org/10.1177/1745691617713052

and family and stay up to date with the happenings and interests of different organizations and communities. Many clubs, hobby groups, and support groups have online forums or social media pages where you can participate in discussions, share experiences, and get advice.

Maintain connections with distant friends and family.

For those with loved ones who live far away, technology can be a lifeline for maintaining relationships. Regularly scheduled video chats, phone calls, or even just exchanging messages through email or social media can help maintain a strong bond with distant friends and family members. Consistent communication through these platforms can provide emotional backing and promote a sense of belongingness.[158]

In addition to one-on-one communication, technology can also facilitate group interactions. You can organize virtual gatherings with family members, friends, or interest groups, allowing everyone to catch up, share experiences, and have fun together. This can be particularly important during special occasions such as holidays, birthdays, or anniversaries

---

[158] Stafford, L., Kline, S. L., & Dimmick, J. (2013). Home e-mail: Relational maintenance and gratification opportunities. Journal of Broadcasting & Electronic Media, 47(4), 589–606. https://doi.org/10.1207/s15506878jobem4704_7

when meeting in person might not be feasible.

To sum up, technology presents numerous prospects for staying socially involved, particularly in situations where physical distance or other constraints make in-person interactions arduous. Men aged 50 and above can foster robust social connections and sustain a lively, gratifying lifestyle by capitalizing on video chats, social media, and online forums.

Building a Support System of Friends & Family:

Connect with People who have Similar Interests or Backgrounds:

Attend events and gatherings.

Building a support system starts with finding people with similar interests, values, or experiences. One way to meet like-minded individuals is by attending events and gatherings related to your hobbies, goods, or cultural background. These events could include social mixers, workshops, cultural festivals, or charity fundraisers. Participating in these activities enables you to converse, exchange ideas, and establish connections with individuals with similar interests or backgrounds.[159]

Engage in conversations and share experiences.

When attending events or gatherings, be open to conversing with others. Share your experiences and listen to the stories of others.

This exchange of ideas and perspectives can foster understanding and camaraderie. Forming significant connections with others can have a constructive effect on your emotional well-being and contribute to a more robust support system.

Reach Out to People You Haven't Spoken to in a While:

Rekindle old friendships.

Over time, it's natural for some friendships to fade as life circumstances change. However, reaching out to friends you haven't spoken to in a while can help rekindle those connections and provide an opportunity for renewed support and companionship. With the aid of social media or other contact information, reach out to old friends to catch up and

[159] Pillemer, K., Munsch, C. L., Fuller-Rowell, T., Riffin, C., & Suitor, J. J. (2015). Ambivalence toward adult children: Differences between mothers and fathers. Journal of Marriage and Family, 77(5), 1109–1125. https://doi.org/10.1111/jomf.12207

reminisce about shared memories. This can fortify existing relationships and add to a more resilient support system.[160]

Reconnect with former colleagues or classmates.

Another way to expand your social network is by reconnecting with former colleagues or classmates. Attending class reunions, alum events, or professional networking gatherings to meet up with people you've lost touch with over the years. Rekindling these connections can result in forming new friendships, exploring professional opportunities, or even rediscovering common interests and hobbies.[161] To maintain good mental and emotional health, men over 50 must build a robust support system of close friends and family. By connecting with individuals with similar interests or backgrounds and re-establishing communication with people from the past, men can establish a solid social network that contributes to a happier, healthier, and more fulfilling life.

---

[160] Rook, K. S. (2015). Social networks in later life: Weighing positive and negative effects on health and well-being. Current Directions in Psychological Science, 24(1), 45–51. https://doi.org/10.1177/0963721414551364

[161] Wrzus, C., Hänel, M., Wagner, J., & Neyer, F. J. (2013). Social network changes and life events across the life span: A meta-analysis. Psychological Bulletin, 139(1), 53–80. https://doi.org/10.1037/a0028601

Spend Time with Family and Friends:

Plan outings and activities together.

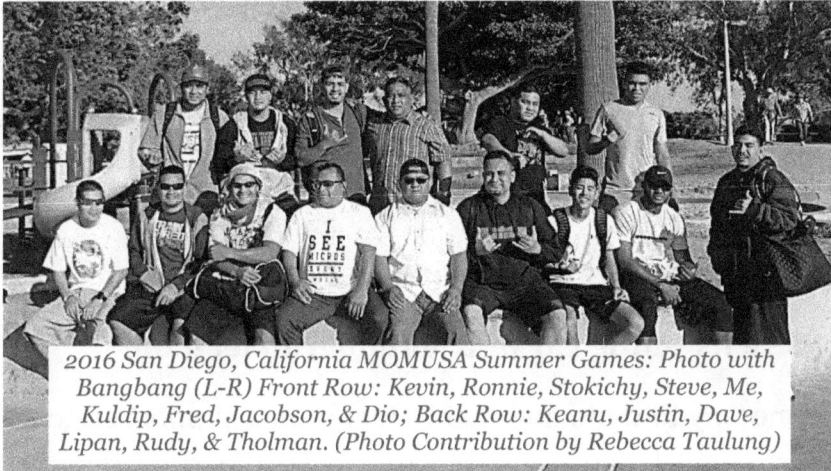

2016 San Diego, California MOMUSA Summer Games: Photo with Bangbang (L-R) Front Row: Kevin, Ronnie, Stokichy, Steve, Me, Kuldip, Fred, Jacobson, & Dio; Back Row: Keanu, Justin, Dave, Lipan, Rudy, & Tholman. (Photo Contribution by Rebecca Taulung)

Quality time with your loved ones and friends is crucial for preserving solid relationships and a dependable support system. Plan outings and activities you can enjoy together, such as family dinners, movie nights, or weekend trips. These gatherings allow bonding, relaxation, and creating shared memories. Participating in group activities or events can also help foster a sense of belonging and promote emotional well-being.[162]

Create lasting memories.

As you engage in activities with family and friends,

---

[162] Greenfield, E. A., & Marks, N. F. (2004). Formal volunteering as a protective factor for older adults' psychological well-being. The Journal of Gerontology,

prioritize forming enduring memories you can treasure for years. Capture special moments through photographs or videos and reminisce about your experiences together. These shared memories can reinforce your bonds with loved ones and foster a sense of continuity and identity within your support system.[163]

Offer Support to Others in Need:

Be a listening ear or a shoulder to lean on

One way to build and maintain a robust support system is by offering support to others when needed. Be a good listener and provide a compassionate, non-judgmental ear for friends and family members who may be going through challenging times. At times, merely being present to listen and empathize with can substantially impact someone's life.

Provide advice or assistance when possible.

When appropriate, offer advice or assistance to those in your support network who may need help. This can include offering practical support, such as helping with household tasks, or emotional support, like encouragement and

---

Series B: Psychological Sciences and Social Sciences, 59(5), S258–S264. https://doi.org/10.1093/geronb/59.5.S258

[163] Alea, N., & Bluck, S. (2007). I'll keep you in mind: The intimacy function of autobiographical memory. Applied Cognitive Psychology, 21(8), 1091–1111. https://doi.org/10.1002/acp.1316

reassurance. By being a reliable source of support for others, you can strengthen your relationships and create a reciprocal environment of care and trust.

Ask for Help When Needed:

Be open about your needs and feelings.

While offering support to others is essential, it's equally important to ask for help when needed. Be open about your feelings, needs, and concerns with your support network. Sharing your thoughts and emotions can ease stress, offer relief, and encourage a deeper connection with others.

Accept support from others graciously.

When friends and family members offer their assistance, accept their support graciously. Remember that asking for help is not a sign of weakness but a natural part of maintaining healthy relationships. By being open to receiving support, you can strengthen your connections and ensure your support system remains solid and reliable.[164]

In summary, dedicating time to loved ones, extending support to those who require it, and being willing to seek help when

---

[164] Cohen, S., & Wills, T. A. (1985). Stress, social support, and the buffering hypothesis. Psychological Bulletin, 98(2), 310–357. https://doi.org/10.1037/0033-2909.98.2.310

necessary is essential in creating and maintaining a support system for men over 50. Through actively fostering and maintaining these connections, men can establish a solid groundwork of love, trust, and care that can contribute to a healthier and more satisfying life. Spending time with family and friends, offering support to others in need, and asking for help when necessary are essential to building and maintaining a support system for men over 50. By actively nurturing these relationships, you can create a foundation of love, trust, and care that will contribute to a healthier, more fulfilling life. By following these strategies for connecting with others and building a strong support system, men over 50 can enjoy a more vibrant social life, enhanced mental and emotional well-being, and improved overall health. Engaging in social activities, staying connected through technology, and seeking out opportunities to support others and ask for help are all essential components of a balanced, active lifestyle for men in their later years.

Encourage Healthy Relationships:

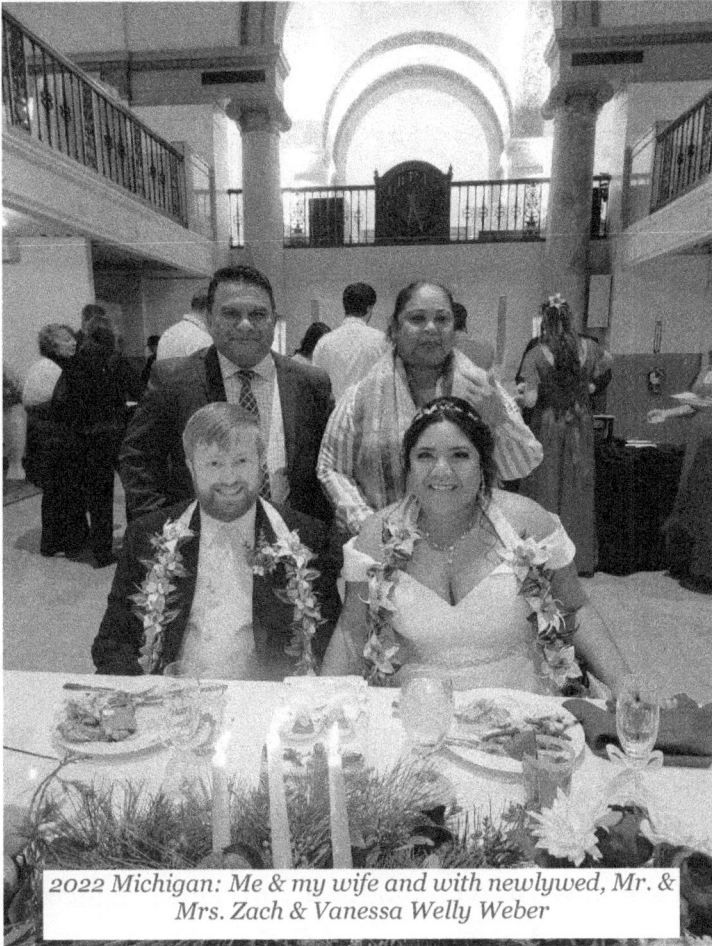

2022 Michigan: Me & my wife and with newlywed, Mr. & Mrs. Zach & Vanessa Welly Weber

Foster open communication and trust.

For men over 50, it is vital to cultivate healthy relationships within their support network. One essential aspect of a healthy relationship is fostering open communication and trust. Engage in honest conversations with friends and family, discussing your feelings, thoughts, and concerns. Active listening and empathy can help build understanding and trust among the people in your support network.[165]

Set boundaries and respect others' boundaries.

Setting boundaries and respecting the boundaries of others is another critical aspect of maintaining healthy relationships. Communicate your limits and preferences and hear about the limitations of others. Respecting personal boundaries helps create a supportive environment where everyone feels valued and respected.[166]

Appreciate Those Around You:

Express Gratitude and Appreciation for Their Presence

It is essential to take a moment to express gratitude and appreciation toward the people in your life who offer you support, kindness, and companionship. This practice can help to fortify your relationships and promote a sense of mutual respect and understanding. Additionally, studies have

---

[165] MacGeorge, E. L., Clark, R. A., & Gillihan, S. J. (2004). Sex differences in the provision of skillful emotional support: The role of evaluation. Communication Reports, 17(2), 87-96. https://doi.org/10.1080/08934210409389385

[166] Beauchamp, M. R., Lemyre, L., & Lalande, D. (2011). Boundary management in sport: Coach–athlete relationships. In S. Jowett & D. Lavallee (Eds.), Social psychology in sport (pp. 229-239). Human Kinetics.

revealed that expressing gratitude can enhance relationship satisfaction and contribute to overall well-being.[167] Therefore, we must understand that cultivating gratitude toward your loved ones can positively affect your relationships and overall well-being.

Celebrate successes and support each other in difficult times.

In your support network, it's essential to celebrate each other's successes and be there for one another during challenging times.

Acknowledge the achievements of your friends and family members and offer your encouragement and support when they face setbacks or difficulties. Demonstrating your concern for good and evil helps nurture solid and lasting relationships.[168]

To conclude, encouraging healthy relationships and appreciating those around you is vital to maintaining a solid support system for men over 50. By fostering open communication and trust, setting and respecting boundaries,

---

[167] Algoe, S. B., Gable, S. L., & Maisel, N. C. (2013). It's the little things: Everyday gratitude as a booster shot for romantic relationships. Personal Relationships, 20(3), 217-233. https://doi.org/10.1111/j.1475-6811.2012.01401.x

[168] Collins, N. L., & Feeney, B. C. (2000). A safe haven: An attachment theory perspective on support seeking and caregiving in intimate relationships. Journal of Personality and Social Psychology, 78(6), 1053-1073. https://doi.org/10.1037/0022-3514.78.6.1053

expressing gratitude, celebrating others' successes, and supporting one another in difficult times, you can create a network of loving, caring, and supportive relationships that contribute to a happier and healthier life.

Key Points Checklist for Chapter 7: Social Health

1. **Prioritize Social Engagement**: Emphasize the importance of staying socially active. Regularly engage in social activities with friends, family, or community members to foster a sense of belonging and improve mood.

2. **Foster Meaningful Connections**: Find opportunities to establish deeper connections with those around you. This could be through joining clubs, volunteering, or exploring new hobbies. Building relationships adds richness to life and enhances mental well-being.

3. **Leverage Technology for Connection**: Utilize technology to stay connected, especially when physical meetings aren't possible. Video chats, social media, and online forums can help maintain social ties and provide a sense of community.

4. **Create a Support System**: Cultivate a network of friends and family who provide emotional support and companionship. To build this system, attend gatherings, share experiences, and reconnect with old friends.

5. **Promote Healthy Relationships**: Encourage open communication, trust, and mutual respect in your relationships. Expressing gratitude and appreciation can strengthen bonds and contribute to overall happiness.

Call to Action:

Now that we've explored the key aspects of maintaining social health, it's time to implement this knowledge. Here's your five-step action plan:

1. **Stay Socially Active**: Commit to engaging in social activities regularly. These interactions are vital for mental well-being and can significantly enhance your quality of life.

2. **Build Meaningful Connections**: Seek out opportunities to connect with others. Join a club, volunteer at a local charity, or take up a new hobby. These activities can provide a sense of purpose and community.

3. **Use Technology to Connect**: Embrace the power of technology to stay connected with friends and family. Virtual meetings can help bridge the gap when physical meetups aren't possible.

4. **Develop Your Support System**: Invest time in building a solid network of friends and family. This support system can provide comfort, advice, and companionship.

5. **Nurture Healthy Relationships**: Prioritize open communication, trust, and respect in all your relationships. Remember, it's the quality of your relationships that contributes to your happiness and well-being.

Your social health is just as important as your physical health. Taking proactive steps and implementing the above checklist can enhance your social well-being and lead a more fulfilling life. So, let's commit to staying socially engaged, fostering healthy relationships, and nurturing a solid support system. Remember, every connection counts!

Chapter 8: Financial Health

"You must gain control over your money, or the lack of it will forever control you."

~ Dave Ramsey

Know-how For Your Future

Retirement Preparation Tips:

Develop a Plan for Retirement:

Creating a detailed retirement plan is crucial for men over 50 to ensure financial stability and a comfortable lifestyle during their post-working years. The following steps outline how to develop an effective retirement plan:

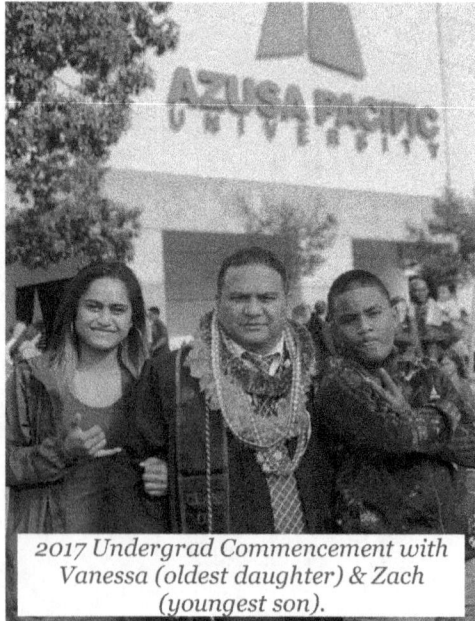

2017 Undergrad Commencement with Vanessa (oldest daughter) & Zach (youngest son).

a. **Estimate retirement expenses**: Begin by projecting your expenses during retirement. Consider costs such as housing, healthcare, utilities, groceries, transportation, insurance, and leisure activities. Additionally, consider any outstanding debts, like mortgages or loans, that must be repaid during retirement. It's essential to factor in inflation, as the cost of living will likely increase over time.

b. **Determine sources of retirement income:** Identify the sources of income you expect to have during retirement. Familiar sources include social security, pensions, investments, annuities, rental income, or part-time employment. Having multiple income streams can provide added financial security during retirement.

c. **Calculate your retirement savings goal:** Compare your projected expenses with your expected income sources to determine the amount you need to save for a comfortable retirement. This calculation will help you set specific savings milestones and develop a plan to reach those targets.

d. **Develop a savings and investment strategy:** Establish a plan for regular contributions to retirement accounts, such as IRAs or 401(k)s.

Additionally, consider other investment options like stocks, bonds, and real estate to diversify your portfolio and potentially increase your returns.

e. **Reassess and adjust your plan periodically:** As you approach retirement, your financial situation, goals, and priorities may change. It is essential to regularly assess and modify your retirement plan to ensure that it continues to meet your present needs and goals. This can entail raising your savings rate, altering your investment approach, or revising your retirement objectives.

f. **Consult with a financial advisor:** Seek professional advice from a financial advisor who can provide personalized guidance and recommendations based on your unique financial situation. An advisor can help you optimize your retirement plan and navigate complex financial decisions.

Research Different Retirement Options:

Understanding various retirement plans and their features can help you choose the best option for your financial situation. Some standard retirement plans include traditional IRAs, Roth IRAs, 401(k)s, and other pension plans. Traditional IRAs offer tax-deductible contributions, but withdrawals during retirement are taxable. While Roth IRAs do not provide contribution tax deductions, they allow for tax-free qualified withdrawals. On the other hand, employer-sponsored plans such as 401(k)s frequently come with employer-matching contributions, which can significantly boost your savings. Although less common today, pensions can provide a steady income stream during retirement based on your years of service and salary history.[169] Assessing these options and their tax implications can help you maximize your retirement savings and minimize your tax burden.

One of our primary goals in the journey towards retirement is to reach the "Zero Income Tax" Bracket. While standard retirement plans may offer tax-free income, an Indexed Universal Life (IUL) policy provides unique benefits that these conventional income streams cannot match. According to David McKnight, IUL offers three distinct advantages:[170]

1. **Long-Term Care Coverage:** One of the standout

---

[169] US News & World Report (2021). Retirement Planning for Men Over 50. Retrieved from: https://money.usnews.com/money/retirement/articles/retirement-planning-for-men-over-50

[170] The Power of Zero, David McKnight. Retrieved from https://www.youtube.com/watch?v=NmbJiAILGLc

benefits of an IUL policy is that it can double as long-term care coverage. If a policyholder cannot perform two out of six essential daily tasks, such as bathing or eating, and their doctor can confirm this, the insurance company can provide them with a check for 25% of the death benefit. This feature acts as a safety net, ensuring you have financial support when you need it most. For example, if your death benefit is $500,000, you could receive $125,000 to cover long-term care costs.

2. **Volatility Shield:** An IUL policy also protects against market volatility. This means that even if the stock market sees significant fluctuations, the cash value of your IUL policy remains stable. For instance, if the market takes a downturn, an IUL policyholder won't see a decrease in their policy's cash value. Knowing your investment is protected from market instability, this stability can provide peace of mind.

3. **Bond Alternative:** Finally, an IUL policy can be an effective alternative to bonds. While bonds are traditionally considered a safe investment option, they may not offer the same growth potential as an IUL policy. By allocating funds to an IUL policy, you could achieve higher returns while still maintaining protection against market volatility. Let's say you have

$100,000 to invest. Putting that money into bonds might result in a 2% return annually. However, with an IUL policy, that return could be much higher, offering you more significant growth potential.

An IUL policy can provide unique benefits, from long-term care coverage to protection against market volatility and the potential for higher returns. It's a financial tool that offers life insurance and a comprehensive wealth accumulation and preservation strategy.

Start Saving for Retirement and Make Regular Contributions:

Thanks to the power of compounding, initiating retirement savings as early as possible and making consistent contributions can lead to significant accumulation over time. Experts recommend saving at least 15% of your income for retirement, although this percentage may vary depending on individual circumstances.[171] One way to maximize your retirement savings is to participate in employer-sponsored plans like 401(k)s, contributing either the maximum allowed amount or at least enough to receive the full employer match. Additionally, consider donating to IRAs and other investment

---

[171] Vision Retirement: 6 Things You Can Do in Your 50s to Better Prepare for Retirement. https://www.visionretirement.com/articles/better-prepare-for-retirement50s

accounts to diversify your retirement savings further. Regularly reviewing and adjusting your contributions based on your financial goals and changing circumstances can help ensure a comfortable retirement.

Consider Reducing Spending to Save More Money:

If you want to boost your retirement savings, it's worth examining your current spending patterns and pinpointing areas where you can reduce your expenses. Focus on eliminating unnecessary costs, such as dining out frequently or multiple streaming subscriptions, and redirect those funds toward retirement savings. Implementing a budget can help you track your expenses and allocate funds more effectively.[172] By reducing spending and prioritizing savings, you can accumulate a more substantial retirement nest egg and ensure a comfortable lifestyle during your post-working years.

Make Use of Employer Benefits such as 401(K)S and other Retirement Funds:

Employer-sponsored retirement plans, such as 401(k)s, are valuable tools for building retirement savings. These plans often include matching employer contributions, significantly

---

[172] Investopedia (2021). What Is a Budget? Retrieved from: https://www.investopedia.com/terms/b/budget.asp

boosting your savings. Be sure to contribute at least enough to receive the full employer match, as not doing so would mean leaving *free money* on the table. In addition to 401(k)s, explore other employer-sponsored benefits that can support your retirement planning, such as pension plans, profit-sharing plans, or employee stock ownership plans (ESOPs). Taking full advantage of these benefits can be crucial in securing your financial future.

Review Social Security Benefits:

Social Security is a vital component of retirement income for many individuals. As you approach retirement, it's essential to understand your expected Social Security benefits and how they fit into your overall retirement plan. The amount you receive depends on your lifetime earnings, the age at which you start claiming benefits, and your marital status. Obtaining an estimate of your future Social Security benefits is possible by accessing your Social Security statement online through the Social Security Administration's website. Delaying the age at which you claim Social Security can result in higher monthly payments, so consider the best time to start receiving benefits based on your financial needs and life expectancy.[173]

Talk to a Financial Advisor for Additional Guidance:

Retirement planning can be complex, and navigating various investment options, tax implications, and other financial decisions can be overwhelming. Getting advice from a financial advisor can be beneficial, as they can offer tailored guidance based on your specific financial situation and goals. They can assist you in optimizing your retirement plan, recommend suitable investment opportunities, and ensure that you're progressing toward meeting your financial objectives. They can advise on estate planning, tax strategies, and other critical financial matters. Engaging the services of a financial advisor can help you feel more confident in your retirement planning decisions and provide peace of mind, knowing you are on the right path.[174]

---

[173] US News & World Report (2021). Retirement Planning for Men Over 50. Retrieved from: https://money.usnews.com/money/retirement/articles/retirement-planning-for-men-over-50

[174] Vision Retirement: 6 Things You Can Do in Your 50s to Better Prepare for Retirement. https://www.visionretirement.com/articles/better-prepare-for-retirement50s

Investing & Saving for the Future.

Create A Budget and Plan Out Your Expenses:

Developing a budget is a crucial step in managing your finances and ensuring you have adequate funds for both short-term expenses and long-term goals, such as retirement. A well-structured budget can help you identify spending patterns, prioritize financial objectives, and allocate resources effectively. The following steps outline how to create a budget and plan your expenses:[175]

a. **Determine your income sources.**

   Begin by calculating your total monthly income, including your salary, investment returns, rental income, or any other sources of revenue. Ensure to account for taxes and other deductions when determining your net income.

b. **List your fixed and variable expenses.**

   Identify all your monthly expenses, dividing them into fixed and variable categories. Fixed expenses are costs that do not change monthly and remain the same throughout the agreed tenure. They include mortgage or rent payments, utilities, insurance

---

[175] Investopedia (2021). What Is a Budget? Retrieved from: https://www.investopedia.com/terms/b/budget.asp

premiums, and loan repayments. Variable expenses, on the other hand, may change from month to month, such as groceries, transportation, entertainment, and dining out.

c. Categorize your expenses.

Organize your expenses into meaningful categories, such as housing, food, transportation, healthcare, and leisure. This organization will help you visualize your spending patterns and identify areas where you may be overspending.

d. Set financial goals.

It's essential to create short-term and long-term financial objectives, such as establishing an emergency fund, saving for a holiday, or contributing to your retirement savings. Clear goals can help you prioritize your spending and allocate your resources more effectively.

e. Allocate your income to each category.

Distribute your income among your expense categories, ensuring you have sufficient funds to cover your fixed costs and contribute to your financial goals. This allocation will serve as a guideline for your monthly spending.

THE AGE OF OPTIMAL HEALTH

f. Track your spending.

Regularly monitor your spending to ensure you stay within the limits established in your budget. Keeping track of your expenses can aid in identifying areas where you may need to modify your spending habits or allocate your funds differently to meet your financial goals.

g. Adjust your budget as needed.

Your financial situation and priorities may change over time, requiring adjustments to your budget. Periodically review and update your budget to ensure it remains aligned with your current needs and objectives. This may involve increasing your savings rate, reallocating funds to different expense categories, or modifying your financial goals.

Creating a budget and planning your expenses can significantly contribute to your financial well-being and provide a solid foundation for achieving your long-term goals, such as a comfortable retirement.

Explore Different Investment Options:

Diversifying your investments is critical to achieving long-term financial success and mitigating risks associated with market fluctuations. By exploring various investment options, you can spread your capital across different assets and sectors, reducing the impact of any single underperforming investment on your overall portfolio. The following investment options can help you build a well-rounded portfolio:

a. Stocks

Shares of stocks represent ownership in a company and have the potential to offer substantial returns over the long run. Investing in stocks provides an opportunity to participate in a company's growth and profits. While stocks can be volatile in the short term, they have historically offered higher returns than bonds or cash over long periods.[176]

b. Bonds.

Bonds are financial instruments governments, corporations, or other entities use to raise funds. Investing in bonds involves lending money to the issuer and receiving interest payments for a specified duration. Bonds typically generate lower returns than

---

[176] Bankrate (2021). Understanding the Basics of Investing. Retrieved from: https://www.bankrate.com/investing/golden-rules-of-investing/

stocks, but they provide a more stable income source and are perceived as being less risky.

c. **Mutual funds and exchange-traded funds (ETFs).**

Mutual funds and ETFs offer a convenient and accessible means of investing in a diversified range of assets, including stocks, bonds, and other investment options. They enable investors to diversify without purchasing individual securities, making them a convenient option for those seeking a diverse investment portfolio. ETFs trade on stock exchanges, offering additional flexibility and liquidity compared to traditional mutual funds.[177]

d. **Real estate.**

Real estate investments can offer income and potential appreciation. Real estate investments can be made directly by purchasing rental units or commercial spaces or indirectly through real estate investment trusts (REITs), companies that own and manage income-producing properties. Real estate

---

1.   [177] Investopedia (2021). What Is Investment Diversification? Retrieved from: https://www.investopedia.com/terms/d/diversification.asp

investments can diversify your portfolio and hedge against inflation.

e. Retirement accounts.

Contributing to tax-advantaged retirement accounts, such as traditional IRAs, Roth IRAs, or 401(k) plans, can offer long-term advantages and enable you to amass wealth for retirement. Depending on the account type, these accounts provide tax benefits, such as tax-deductible contributions or tax-free withdrawals.[178]

f. Commodities and precious metals.

Investing in commodities like oil, gold, or agricultural products can diversify your portfolio and safeguard against inflation or economic uncertainty. One way to invest in things is by purchasing futures contracts, while another is through indirect investment via mutual funds or ETFs focusing on commodities or precious metals.

g. Alternative investments.

Certain investors may aim to expand their portfolio's diversification by investing in alternative assets like

---

[178] US News & World Report (2021). Retirement Planning for Men Over 50. Retrieved from: https://money.usnews.com

private equity, venture capital, or hedge funds. Although these investments have the potential to yield high returns, they also tend to involve higher risks and may not be appropriate for all investors.

Before investing, assessing your financial goals, risk tolerance, and investment horizon is essential. Consulting with a financial advisor can help you determine which investment options best suit your needs and develop a diversified portfolio that aligns with your objectives.

Determine the Amount of Risk You are Willing to Take on with Investments.

Risk tolerance refers to an investor's ability and willingness to accept fluctuations in the value of their investments. Understanding your risk tolerance is critical when building your investment portfolio, as it helps you select the appropriate mix of assets that align with your financial goals and comfort level. To assess your risk tolerance, consider the following factors:

a. Investment horizon.

The length of time you plan to hold an investment before needing to access the funds is known as your investment horizon. Longer horizons generally allow for greater risk-taking, as you have more time to recover from potential losses. Conversely, shorter horizons require a more conservative approach to minimize the likelihood of significant losses.

b. Financial goals.

Your investment objectives should inform your risk tolerance. If you have ambitious financial goals that require high returns, you may need to assume higher risks. However, a lower-risk approach may be more appropriate if your goals are more modest or focused on preserving capital.

c. Personal financial situation.

Consider your current financial situation, including your income, expenses, debt, and emergency savings. You may be more comfortable taking on higher-risk investments with a stable income, minimal debt, and a robust emergency fund. On the other hand, if you have financial obligations or limited savings, a more conservative approach may be necessary.

d. Emotional comfort.

Your emotional comfort with market fluctuations is crucial to risk tolerance. Some investors are more risk-averse and may become anxious during market volatility, while others are more comfortable with the ups and downs of the market. Understanding your emotional reactions to investment risk and building a portfolio that allows you to sleep well at night is essential.

Diversify your Portfolio and Spread Investments Across Different Sectors

Diversification is a crucial investment principle that distributes your investments among various asset classes, sectors, and geographic regions. This strategy is beneficial in reducing the overall risk of your portfolio, as losses in one investment can be offset by gains in another. The following tips can help you diversify your portfolio effectively:

a. **Invest in different asset classes.**

Allocate your investments among stocks, bonds, and other asset classes, such as real estate or commodities. Each asset class has unique characteristics and may perform differently under varying market conditions. Investing in multiple asset classes can reduce the impact of any underperforming investment on your overall portfolio.

b. **Invest in various sectors and industries.**

Invest in a mix of sectors and industries within each asset class. For example, diversify your stock holdings across technology, healthcare, financial services, and consumer goods sectors. This strategy helps minimize sector-specific risks and ensures your investments are not overly concentrated in one area.

c. Invest globally.

Diversify your investments across different geographic regions to reduce exposure to country-specific risks, such as political instability, currency fluctuations, or economic downturns. Global diversification can also provide access to growth opportunities in emerging markets and help protect your portfolio from regional economic downturns.

d. Rebalance your portfolio periodically.

As time passes, changes in the market can cause your asset allocation to change, leading to an investment portfolio that no longer corresponds with your risk tolerance and financial objectives. Regularly rebalancing your portfolio—selling overweight assets and buying underweight assets—can help maintain your desired asset allocation and ensure your investments remain diversified.

e. Consider professional help.

If you're unsure how to diversify your portfolio effectively, consult a financial advisor. Financial experts can offer personalized guidance considering your investment horizon, risk tolerance, and financial objectives. With their help, you can construct and manage a well-diversified investment portfolio.

Diversification does not guarantee profits or eliminate the risk of loss, but it is a proven strategy for managing investment risk and optimizing long-term returns. Distributing your investments among various asset classes, sectors, and geographic regions can decrease the impact of market fluctuations and enhance the likelihood of fulfilling your financial objectives.[179]

Determining the amount of risk, you are willing to take with investments and diversifying your portfolio across different sectors is essential to building a solid financial foundation. Understanding your risk tolerance and implementing a diversified investment strategy can help you minimize risk, optimize returns, and achieve your financial goals. It's crucial to regularly review and adjust your investment strategy as needed, and seeking professional guidance from a financial

---

[179] Investopedia (2021). What Is Investment Diversification? Retrieved from: https://www.investopedia.com/terms/d/diversification.asp

advisor can be invaluable in navigating the complex world of investing.

Put Aside Emergency Savings to Cover Unexpected Expenses:

Establishing an emergency fund is crucial to financial planning, as it provides a safety net to cover unexpected expenses or income disruptions. Life is unpredictable; unforeseen medical emergencies, job losses, or costly home repairs can quickly derail your financial stability. By building an emergency fund, you can better manage these challenges without incurring debt or compromising your long-term financial goals.[180]

It is generally advised by financial professionals to save up to three to six months' worth of living expenses in an emergency fund. However, the optimal amount can vary depending on your financial circumstances, job stability, and risk tolerance. To build your emergency fund, consider the following tips:

1. **Start small and set realistic goals.**

   If saving several months' worth of expenses seems daunting, begin with a smaller, more achievable

---

[180] Investopedia (2021). What Is an Emergency Fund? Retrieved from: https://www.investopedia.com/terms/e/emergency_fund.asp

target. Aim to initially save $1,000- or one month's worth of living expenses, and gradually increase your savings goal as you build momentum.

2. **Make saving automatic.**

One helpful method is to set up recurring transfers from your checking account to a dedicated savings account every month. This method ensures that you keep consistently and reduces the temptation to use the money for non-essential purchases.

3. **Adjust your budget and cut expenses.**

Review your budget and identify areas where you can reduce spending. Redirecting funds from discretionary costs, such as dining out or entertainment, toward your emergency fund can help you reach your savings goal more quickly.

4. **Find additional sources of income.**

If possible, consider taking on a part-time job, freelance work, or side hustle to supplement your income and accelerate your emergency fund savings.

Review Your Investment Strategy Periodically and Adjust as Needed:

Your financial goals, risk tolerance, and investment horizon may change as you progress through different life stages. Regularly reviewing your investment strategy and adjusting as needed can help ensure your portfolio remains aligned with your evolving needs.[181]

To effectively review and adjust your investment strategy, consider the following steps:

a. Reevaluate your financial goals.

Assess whether your financial objectives have changed since you last reviewed your investment strategy. This evaluation may include updating your retirement savings target, adjusting your investment horizon, or modifying your risk tolerance.

b. Analyze your portfolio performance.

Review the performance of your investments, comparing their returns to relevant benchmarks or market indices. This analysis can help you identify

---

1.   [181] Bankrate (2021). Understanding the Basics of Investing. Retrieved from: https://www.bankrate.com/investing/golden-rules-of-investing/

underperforming assets and determine whether adjustments are necessary.

c. Rebalance your portfolio.

If your asset allocation has drifted from your target due to market fluctuations, rebalance your portfolio by selling overweight and underweight assets. Rebalancing helps maintain your desired risk level and ensures your investments remain diversified.

d. Review your investment fees.

High fees can erode your investment returns over time. Regularly review the costs associated with your investments, such as expense ratios for mutual funds or ETFs, and consider switching to lower-cost options if appropriate.

e. Consult with a financial advisor.

If you're uncertain how to modify your investment approach or require guidance on intricate financial matters, seek advice from a financial advisor. These professionals can provide personalized advice based on your unique financial situation and goals, helping you navigate the ever-changing investment landscape.

Regularly reviewing and adjusting your investment strategy is essential for staying on track toward your financial goals and adapting to changes in your circumstances or the broader market environment.

Remember, putting aside emergency savings to cover unexpected expenses and periodically reviewing your investment strategy are critical components of a sound financial plan. An emergency fund acts as a financial safety net, enabling you to handle unexpected obstacles without taking on debt or jeopardizing your long-term goals. Regularly evaluating and adjusting your investment strategy ensures that your portfolio stays aligned with your evolving needs and helps you achieve your financial objectives.

Integrating these strategies into your financial plan can establish a stable financial security and success base. It is crucial to continuously monitor your investments, keep abreast of market developments, and contemplate seeking expert advice from a financial advisor to navigate the intricate world of investing. Adopting a proactive stance toward managing your finances allows you to position yourself for a prosperous future and experience peace of mind from financial stability.

Track your Investments and Monitor Performance Regularly:

To maintain a healthy investment portfolio and achieve your financial goals, tracking your investments and monitoring their performance actively is essential. Regular monitoring lets you identify potential issues early on, make timely adjustments, and optimize your investment strategy.[182] Consider the following tips for tracking your investments and monitoring their performance:

a. Set up a tracking system.

Develop a system for tracking your investments that works best for you. This system can be as simple as a spreadsheet or as advanced as specialized investment tracking software. Maintaining an organized and up-to-date record of your investments, including the purchase date, cost basis, current value, and performance, is critical.

b. Establish a review schedule.

Determine how often you'll review your investments, such as monthly, quarterly, or annually. The frequency of your review may depend on the type of

---

[182] Bankrate (2021). Understanding the Basics of Investing. Retrieved from: https://www.bankrate.com/investing/golden-rules-of-investing/

investments you hold, your investment horizon, and your personal preferences. Regularly reviewing your assets ensures you stay informed about their performance and can react quickly to changes in the market.

c. Stay informed about market trends and news.

Keep abreast of financial information and directions that may impact on your investments. Understanding the broader market context can help you make more informed investment decisions and better anticipate changes in your portfolio's performance.

d. Review your investment objectives and risk tolerance.

As you monitor your investments, periodically reassess your financial goals and risk tolerance to ensure they align with your investment strategy. Adjust your plan as needed to reflect changes in your circumstances or the market environment.

Talk To a Financial Advisor for Additional Guidance

While taking ownership of your financial future is essential, seeking professional guidance from a financial advisor can be invaluable in navigating the complex investing world. A financial advisor can help you with the following:

a. Develop a comprehensive financial plan.

A financial advisor can work with you to create a personalized financial plan that considers your unique goals, risk tolerance, and investment horizon. This plan serves as a roadmap for achieving your financial objectives and provides a framework for making informed investment decisions.

b. Identify suitable investment options.

Based on your financial plan, a financial advisor can recommend appropriate investment vehicles that align with your goals, risk tolerance, and investment horizon. These recommendations may include individual stocks, bonds, mutual funds, ETFs, or alternative investments.

c. Implement a diversified investment strategy.

A financial advisor can help you build and maintain a well-diversified portfolio that spreads your investments across various asset classes, sectors, and geographic regions. Diversification reduces the impact of market fluctuations and helps optimize long-term returns.

d. Monitor and adjust your investment strategy.

A financial advisor can regularly review your investment portfolio, assess its performance, and recommend adjustments. This oversight ensures your investments align with your financial goals and market conditions.

Guide on complex financial matters:

Financial advisors can offer expert advice on complex financial topics, such as tax-efficient investing, estate planning, or retirement income strategies. This guidance can help you make well-informed decisions and optimize your economic outcomes. Tracking your investments, monitoring their performance regularly, and seeking advice from a financial advisor are essential components of a successful financial plan. You can make more informed decisions and optimize your investment strategy by staying informed about your assets and the broader market environment. Additionally, a financial advisor can provide valuable insights, expertise, and personalized advice to help you navigate the complex investing world and achieve your financial goals.

You can build a solid financial success and security foundation by actively monitoring your investments and seeking professional guidance. Remember that your financial plan should be changed and evolve as your circumstances, financial goals, and the market environment change.

Being proactive in managing your finances and staying informed about market trends can empower you to make well-informed investment decisions and maximize your financial potential. Ultimately, taking control of your financial future and adopting a disciplined approach to investing can help you secure a comfortable retirement and enjoy peace of mind with financial stability.

In summary, the importance of financial planning and retirement preparation for men over 50 cannot be overstated. By developing a comprehensive financial plan, exploring various investment options, creating a diversified portfolio,

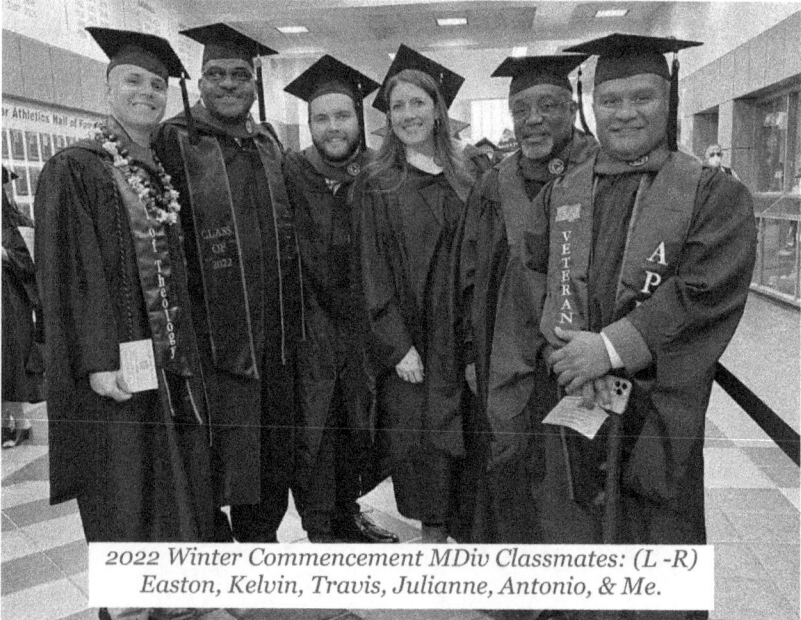

2022 Winter Commencement MDiv Classmates: (L -R) Easton, Kelvin, Travis, Julianne, Antonio, & Me.

and seeking professional guidance, you can set yourself up for a prosperous future. Taking charge of your financial well-being and making informed decisions is essential to ensure you can enjoy a fulfilling and financially secure retirement.

Key Points Checklist for Chapter 8: Financial Health

1. **Estimate Retirement Expenses**: Consider your current lifestyle, future healthcare needs, and inflation when estimating your retirement expenses. This will give you a clear picture of the amount you need to save.

2. **Identify Income Sources**: Consider your potential sources of income in retirement. This could include savings, investments, pensions, or social security. It's wise to have multiple income streams for financial stability.

3. **Set Savings Goals**: Calculate your retirement savings goal and set specific milestones. This will help you stay on track and save enough to support your retirement lifestyle.

4. **Create a Savings Strategy**: Develop an adequate savings and investment strategy. Regular contributions to retirement accounts and diversifying your portfolio can significantly increase your retirement fund.

5. **Revisit Your Plan**: Periodically reassess your retirement plan and make necessary adjustments. A financial advisor can provide personalized guidance and help you optimize your strategy.

Call to Action:

Now that we've outlined the key aspects of financial health, it's time to implement this knowledge. Here's your five-step action plan:

1. **Start Saving Now**: Time is your biggest ally when saving for retirement. Start making regular

contributions now, aiming to save at least 15% of your income.

2. **Cut Unnecessary Spending**: Implement a budget and reduce unnecessary costs. Every dollar saved today can contribute significantly to your retirement fund.

3. **Leverage Employer Benefits**: If available, take full advantage of employer benefits such as 401(k) matching contributions. This is essentially 'free money' that can boost your retirement savings.

4. **Understand Social Security Benefits**: Review your expected Social Security benefits and consider the best time to start receiving them. This decision can impact your overall retirement income.

5. **Seek Professional Advice**: Consult with a financial advisor for personalized retirement planning and investment strategies guidance. Their expertise can be invaluable in securing your financial future.

Financial health is crucial for a stress-free and comfortable retirement. You can ensure a financially secure future by implementing this checklist and taking proactive steps today. So, let's commit to saving wisely, investing strategically, and planning meticulously for our retirement years. Remember, every dollar saved today is a step towards a financially secure tomorrow!

Conclusion

Reflecting on my journey as a Micronesian establishing residence in the United States, I am grateful for the wealth of knowledge and insights I have gathered. Each chapter in my book, "The Age of Optimal Health: A Comprehensive Guide for Men Over 50 to Maintain an Active Lifestyle, Ensure Proper Nutrition, and Take Preventative Measures," has been instrumental in shaping my understanding of health, wellness, and lifestyle, guiding me towards a more fulfilling

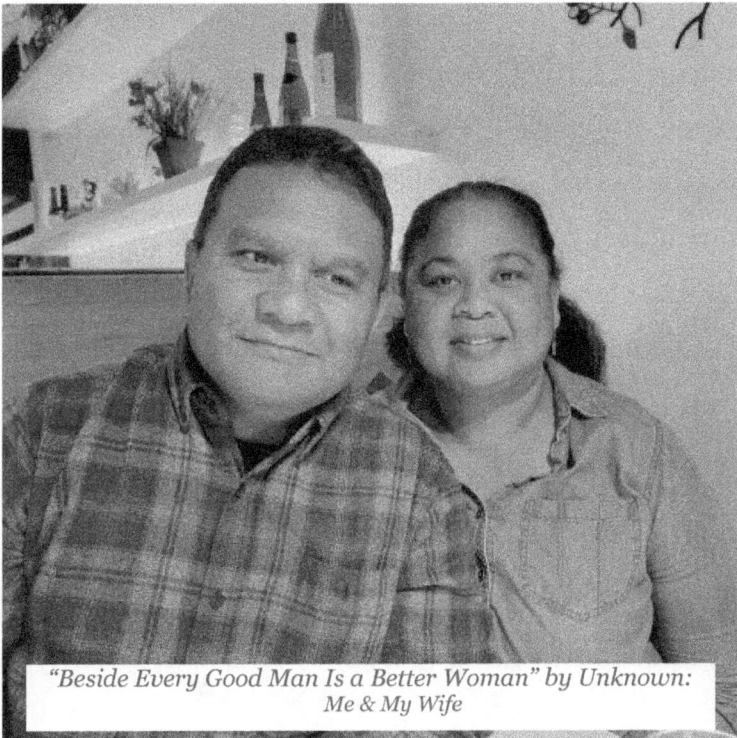

"Beside Every Good Man Is a Better Woman" by Unknown: Me & My Wife

and prosperous life.

In the introduction, I set the stage for prioritizing health at every stage of life. It was here that I emphasized the need for sustainable physical activity and the profound impact it can have on our overall well-being.

Chapter 1 delved into the nuanced realm of stress management. It was a reminder that stress, though a standard part of life, needs to be managed effectively. Stress can be mitigated through exercise, meditation, and a robust support system, fostering resilience and growth.

Chapter 2 provided an in-depth examination of obesity, exploring its causes, risks, and management strategies. It emphasizes the significant physical and mental health implications of obesity, including cardiovascular diseases, type 2 diabetes, and certain cancers. It underscored the need for comprehensive interventions to address this global health concern.

Chapter 3 underscored the significance of maintaining an active lifestyle for optimal health. Highlighting various physical activities like Tai Chi, yoga, Pilates, cycling, swimming, and running elucidates their beneficial effects on cardiovascular health, weight management, stress reduction, and overall well-being.

Chapter 4 highlighted the importance of regular health screenings for men over 50, such as blood pressure and cholesterol tests, PSA screening, colon and skin cancer screenings, and diabetes screenings. Each step is pivotal in detecting and managing conditions that could lead to severe complications.

Chapter 5 offered a comprehensive overview of Erectile Dysfunction (ED), a condition often overlooked in men's health discourse. It underscored the various physical and psychological factors linked to ED, stressing the importance of acknowledging and addressing this issue for improved health and overall well-being.

Chapter 6 delved into the core elements of sustaining mental well-being, stressing the importance of effective stress management, building a reliable support network, and time management. It underscored the transformative power of engaging in flexibility-promoting activities and aerobic exercises like cycling, swimming, and running in enhancing mental health.

Chapter 7 highlighted the profound importance of nurturing a robust social network, engaging in meaningful relationships, and participating in social activities for overall wellness. This chapter passionately underscored these aspects' pivotal role in providing emotional support, reducing stress, and elevating one's quality of life.

Chapter 8 underscored the critical importance of strategic planning for financial wellness. It emphasizes creating a budget, establishing a retirement plan, diversifying investments, and seeking professional advice to ensure a secure financial future. This chapter is a beacon of guidance for sound financial practices and preparedness.

In conclusion, my journey as a Micronesian in the US has been marked by countless learnings. The knowledge gleaned from each chapter underscores the importance of holistic health - physical, mental, and emotional. By prioritizing these aspects, we pave the way for healthier, happier, and prosperous lives.

I am committed to sharing this knowledge and empowering them to take charge of their health and wellness. Together, we can build a resilient and thriving community. Here's to our collective journey of growth, well-being, and prosperity!

References

1. (2022), Tai chis, Pilates and Yoga, NHS inform Retrieved from: https://www.nhsinform.scot/healthy-living/keeping-active/activities/tai-chi-pilates-and-yoga

2. (2023), Aerobic exercise, Cleveland Clinic Retrieved from: https://my.clevelandclinic.org/health/articles/7050-aerobic-exercise

3. This is the Exact Age When the Average Person Is Most Confident, The Healthy, Retrieved from: https://www.thehealthy.com/mental-health/self-care/age-when-average-person-most-confident/

4. (2013), Cycling - health benefits, Better Health Channel Retrieved from: https://www.betterhealth.vic.gov.au/health/healthyliving/cycling-health-benefits

5. (2013), Swimming – Health Benefits, Better Health Channel Retrieved from:
    https://www.betterhealth.vic.gov.au/health/healthyliving/swimming-health-benefits

6. (2021), 8 Running Benefits for your Body, Brain, and Well-Being, Cigna Healthcare Retrieved from: https://www.cigna.com/knowledge-center/mental-health-benefits-of-running#:~:text=Cardiovascular%20exercise%20can%20create%20new,%2C%20higher%20thinking%2C%20and%20learning.

7. Staying Healthy, Harvard Health Publishing, Harvard Medical School Retrieved from: https://www.health.harvard.edu/category/staying-healthy

8. Physical Activity, World Health Organization Retrieved from: https://www.who.int/health-topics/physical-activity#tab=tab_1

9. (2022), Low Testosterone (Male Hypogonadism), Cleveland Clinic Retrieved from: https://my.clevelandclinic.org/health/diseases/15603-low-testosterone-male-hypogonadism#:~:text=Low%20testosterone%20(male%20hypogonadism)%20is,treatable%20with%20testosterone%20replacement%20therapy.

10. (2023), The hormones that drive male fertility, Legacy Retrieved from: https://www.givelegacy.com/resources/the-hormones-that-drive-male-fertility/

11. Osteoporosis, Causes, NHS Retrieved from: https://www.nhs.uk/conditions/osteoporosis/causes/#:~:text=too%20mu ch%20dieting-,Men,with%20low%20levels%20of%20testosterone.

12. Daniel Yetman (2022), Is there a link between Testosterone level and osteoporosis, Healthline Retrieved from: https://www.healthline.com/health/testosterone-and-osteoporosis

13. Older Adults and Mental Health, Mental Health Information (National Institute of Mental Health) Retrieved from: https://www.nimh.nih.gov/health/topics/older-adults-and-mental-health

14. Exercise: 7 benefits of regular physical activity, Mayo Clinic Retrieved from: https://www.mayoclinic.org/healthy-lifestyle/fitness/in-depth/exercise/art-20048389

15. Warburton, D. E., Nicol, C. W., & Bredin, S. S. (2006). Health benefits of physical activity: the evidence. *CMAJ : Canadian Medical Association journal = journal de l'Association medicale canadienne, 174*(6), 801–809. https://doi.org/10.1503/cmaj.051351

16. Peterson, M. D., Rhea, M. R., & Alvar, B. A. (2005). Applications of the dose-response for muscular strength development: a review of meta-analytic efficacy and reliability for designing training prescription. *Journal of strength and conditioning research, 19*(4), 950–958. https://doi.org/10.1519/R-16874.1

17. Liguori, G., & American College of Sports Medicine. (2020). *ACSM's guidelines for exercise testing and prescription.* Lippincott Williams & Wilkins.

18. US, D. (2004). Bone health and osteoporosis: A Report of the Surgeon General. *http://www. surgeongeneral. gov/library/bonehealth/content. html.*

19. **Bouvard, V., Loomis, D., Guyton, K. Z., Grosse, Y., El Ghissassi, F., Benbrahim-Tallaa, L., ... & Straif, K. (2015). Carcinogenicity of consumption of red and processed meat. *The Lancet Oncology, 16*(16), 1599-1600.**

20. Rodriguez, N. R., DiMarco, N. M., & Langley, S. (2009). Position of the American Dietetic Association, Dietitians of Canada, and the American College of Sports Medicine: Nutrition and athletic performance. *Journal of the American Dietetic Association, 109*(3), 509-527.

21. Paniagua, J. A., Gallego de la Sacristana, A., Romero, I., Vidal-Puig, A.,

Latre, J. M., Sanchez, E., Perez-Martinez, P., Lopez-Miranda, J., & Perez-Jimenez, F. (2007). Monounsaturated fat-rich diet prevents central body fat distribution and decreases postprandial adiponectin expression induced by a carbohydrate-rich diet in insulin-resistant subjects. *Diabetes care, 30*(7), 1717–1723. https://doi.org/10.2337/dc06-2220

22. Mandolesi, L., Polverino, A., Montuori, S., Foti, F., Ferraioli, G., Sorrentino, P., & Sorrentino, G. (2018). Effects of Physical Exercise on Cognitive Functioning and Wellbeing: Biological and Psychological Benefits. *Frontiers in Psychology, 9,* 509. https://doi.org/10.3389/fpsyg.2018.00509

23. Kredlow, M. A., Capozzoli, M. C., Hearon, B. A., Calkins, A. W., & Otto, M. W. (2015). The effects of physical activity on sleep: a meta-analytic review. *Journal of behavioral medicine, 38*(3), 427–449. https://doi.org/10.1007/s10865-015-9617-6

24. American Cancer Society. (2021). Key statistics for prostate cancer. Retrieved from https://www.cancer.org/cancer/prostate-cancer/about/key-statistics.html

25. Mayo Clinic. (2021). Prostate Cancer Screening. Retrieved from https://www.mayoclinic.org/tests-procedures/index?letter=P

26. Radiological Society of North America. (2021). Prostate/Transrectal Ultrasound. Retrieved from https://www.radiologyinfo.org/en/info/prostate-trus

27. American Cancer Society. (2021). American Cancer Society Guideline for Colorectal Cancer Screening. Retrieved from https://www.cancer.org/cancer/colon-rectal-cancer/detection-diagnosis-staging/acs-recommendations.html

28. American Cancer Society. (2021). Skin Cancer Prevention and Early Detection. Retrieved from https://www.cancer.org/cancer/skin-cancer/prevention-and-early-detection.html

29. American Heart Association. (2021). How to Help Prevent Heart Disease At Any Age. Retrieved from https://www.heart.org/en/healthy-living/healthy-lifestyle/how-to-help-prevent-heart-disease-at-any-age

30. Centers for Disease Control and Prevention. (2020). Diabetes Tests. Retrieved from https://www.cdc.gov/diabetes/basics/getting-tested.html

31. National Eye Institute. (2019). Get a Dilated Eye Exam. Retrieved from https://www.nei.nih.gov/learn-about-eye-health/healthy-vision/get-dilated-eye-exam

32. National Osteoporosis Foundation. (n.d.). Bone Density Exam/Testing. Retrieved from https://www.nof.org/patients/diagnosis-information/bone-density-examtesting/

33. National Institute of Mental Health. (2021). Help for Mental Illnesses. Retrieved from https://www.nimh.nih.gov/health/find-help

34. Biddle, S. J. H. (2016). Physical activity and mental health: evidence is growing. World Psychiatry, 15(2), 176-177. https://doi.org/10.1002/wps.20331

35. Goyal, M., Singh, S., Sibinga, E. M., Gould, N. F., Rowland-Seymour, A., Sharma, R., ... & Haythornthwaite, J. A. (2014). Meditation programs for psychological stress and well-being: a systematic review and meta-analysis. JAMA Internal Medicine, 174(3), 357-368. https://doi.org/10.1001/jamainternmed.2013.13018

36. Hofmann, S. G., Asnaani, A., Vonk, I. J., Sawyer, A. T., & Fang, A. (2012). The efficacy of cognitive behavioral therapy: A review of meta-analyses. *Cognitive therapy and research*, 36, 427-440.

37. Lassale, C., Batty, G. D., Baghdadli, A., Jacka, F., Sánchez-Villegas, A., Kivimäki, M., & Akbaraly, T. (2019). Healthy dietary indices and risk of depressive outcomes: a systematic review and meta-analysis of observational studies. Molecular Psychiatry, 24(7), 965-986. https://doi.org/10.1038/s41380-018-0237-8

38. American Psychological Association. (2021). Stress Management. Retrieved from: https://www.apa.org/topics/stress

39. Hofmann, S. G., Asnaani, A., Vonk, I. J., Sawyer, A. T., & Fang, A. (2012). The efficacy of cognitive-behavioral therapy: A review of meta-analyses.

40. Kok, B. E., Coffey, K. A., Cohn, M. A., Catalino, L. I., Vacharkulksemsuk, T., Algoe, S. B., ... & Fredrickson, B. L. (2013). How positive emotions build physical health: Perceived positive social connections account for the upward spiral between positive emotions and vagal tone. Psychological Science, 24(7), 1123-1132. https://doi.org/10.1177/0956797612470827

41. Neff, K. D., & Germer, C. K. (2013). A pilot study and randomized controlled trial of the mindful self-compassion program. Journal of Clinical Psychology, 69(1), 28-44. https://doi.org/10.1002/jclp.21923

42. Pascoe, M. C., & Bauer, I. E. (2015). A systematic review of randomised control trials on the effects of yoga on stress measures and mood. Journal of Psychiatric Research, 68, 270-282. https://doi.org/10.1016/j.jpsychires.2015.07.013

43. Frost, J., & McKelvie, S. (2014). Self-esteem and body satisfaction in male and female elementary school, high school, and university students. Sex Roles, 71(1-2), 45-54. https://doi.org/10.1007/s11199-014-0341-3

44. National Institute on Aging. (2020). Tips to boost your health as you age. U.S. Department of Health and Human Services. Retrieved from https://www.nia.nih.gov/health/infographics/tips-boost-your-health-you-age

45. Cohen, S., Doyle, W. J., Skoner, D. P., Rabin, B. S., & Gwaltney, J. M., Jr (1997). Social ties and susceptibility to the common cold. JAMA, 277(24), 1940-1944. https://doi.org/10.1001/jama.1997.03540480040036

46. Holt-Lunstad, J., Smith, T. B., & Layton, J. B. (2010). Social relationships and mortality risk: A meta-analytic review. PLoS Medicine, 7(7), e1000316. https://doi.org/10.1371/journal.pmed.1000316

47. National Institute on Aging. (2021). Staying connected. U.S. Department of Health and Human Services. https://www.nia.nih.gov/health/staying-connected

48. Holt-Lunstad, J. (2017). The potential public health relevance of social isolation and loneliness: Prevalence, epidemiology, and risk factors.

Public Policy & Aging Report, 27(4), 127-130. https://doi.org/10.1093/ppar/prx030

49. Thoits, P. A., & Hewitt, L. N. (2001). Volunteer work and well-being. Journal of Health and Social Behavior, 42(2), 115-131. https://doi.org/10.2307/3090173

50. Park, D. C., Lodi-Smith, J., Drew, L., Haber, S., Hebrank, A., Bischof, G. N., & Aamodt, W. (2014). The impact of sustained engagement on cognitive function in older adults: The Synapse Project. Psychological Science, 25(1), 103-112. https://doi.org/10.1177/0956797613499592

51. Nowland, R., Necka, E. A., & Cacioppo, J. T. (2018). Loneliness and social internet use: Pathways to reconnection in a digital world? erspectives on Psychological Science, 13(1), 70-87. https://doi.org/10.1177/1745691617713052

52. Stafford, L., Kline, S. L., & Dimmick, J. (2013). Home e-mail: Relational maintenance and gratification opportunities. Journal of Broadcasting & Electronic Media, 47(4), 589-606. https://doi.org/10.1207/s15506878jobem4704_7

53. Pillemer, K., Munsch, C. L., Fuller-Rowell, T., Riffin, C., & Suitor, J. J. (2015). Ambivalence toward adult children: Differences between mothers and fathers. Journal of Marriage and Family, 77(5), 1109-1125. https://doi.org/10.1111/jomf.12207

54. Rook, K. S. (2015). Social networks in later life: Weighing positive and negative effects on health and well-being. Current Directions in Psychological Science, 24(1), 45-51. https://doi.org/10.1177/0963721414551364

55. Wrzus, C., Hänel, M., Wagner, J., & Neyer, F. J. (2013). Social network changes and life events across the life span: A meta-analysis. Psychological Bulletin, 139(1), 53-80. https://doi.org/10.1037/a0028601

56. Greenfield, E. A., & Marks, N. F. (2004). Formal volunteering as a protective factor for older adults' psychological well-being. The Journal of Gerontology, Series B: Psychological Sciences and Social Sciences, 59(5), S258-S264. https://doi.org/10.1093/geronb/59.5.S258

57. Alea, N., & Bluck, S. (2007). I'll keep you in mind: The intimacy function of autobiographical memory. Applied Cognitive Psychology, 21(8), 1091-1111. https://doi.org/10.1002/acp.1316

58. Cohen, S., & Wills, T. A. (1985). Stress, social support, and the buffering hypothesis. Psychological Bulletin, 98(2), 310-357. https://doi.org/10.1037/0033-2909.98.2.310

59. MacGeorge, E. L., Clark, R. A., & Gillihan, S. J. (2004). Sex differences in the provision of skillful emotional support: The role of evaluation. Communication Reports, 17(2), 87-96. https://doi.org/10.1080/08934210409389385

60. Beauchamp, M. R., Lemyre, L., & Lalande, D. (2011). Boundary management in sport: Coach–athlete relationships. In S. Jowett & D. Lavallee (Eds.), Social psychology in sport (pp. 229-239). Human Kinetics.

61. Algoe, S. B., Gable, S. L., & Maisel, N. C. (2013). It's the little things: Everyday gratitude as a booster shot for romantic relationships. Personal Relationships, 20(3), 217-233. https://doi.org/10.1111/j.1475-6811.2012.01401.x

62. Collins, N. L., & Feeney, B. C. (2000). A safe haven: An attachment theory perspective on support seeking and caregiving in intimate relationships. Journal of Personality and Social Psychology, 78(6), 1053-1073. https://doi.org/10.1037/0022-3514.78.6.1053

63. US News & World Report (2021). Retirement Planning for Men Over 50. Retrieved from: https://money.usnews.com/money/retirement/articles/retirement-planning-for-men-over-50

64. Vision Retirement: 6 Things You Can Do in Your 50s to Better Prepare for Retirement. https://www.visionretirement.com/articles/better-prepare-for-retirement50s

65. Investopedia (2021). What Is a Budget? Retrieved from: https://www.investopedia.com/terms/b/budget.asp

66. US News & World Report (2021). Retirement Planning for Men Over 50. Retrieved from: https://money.usnews.com/money/retirement/articles/retirement-planning-for-men-over-50

67. Vision Retirement: 6 Things You Can Do in Your 50s to Better Prepare for Retirement. https://www.visionretirement.com/articles/better-prepare-for-retirement50s

68. Investopedia (2021). What Is a Budget? Retrieved from: https://www.investopedia.com/terms/b/budget.asp

69. Bankrate (2021). Understanding the Basics of Investing. Retrieved from: https://www.bankrate.com/investing/golden-rules-of-investing/

70. Investopedia (2021). What Is Investment Diversification? Retrieved from: https://www.investopedia.com/terms/d/diversification.asp

71. US News & World Report (2021). Retirement Planning for Men Over 50. Retrieved from: https://money.usnews.com

72. Investopedia (2021). What Is Investment Diversification? Retrieved from: https://www.investopedia.com/terms/d/diversification.asp

73. Investopedia (2021). What Is an Emergency Fund? Retrieved from: https://www.investopedia.com/terms/e/emergency_fund.asp

74. Bankrate (2021). Understanding the Basics of Investing. Retrieved from: https://www.bankrate.com/investing/golden-rules-of-investing/

75. Bankrate (2021). Understanding the Basics of Investing. Retrieved from: https://www.bankrate.com/investing/golden-rules-of-investing/

76. Harvard T.H. Chan School of Public Health. (n.d.). The Nutrition Source. https://www.hsph.harvard.edu/nutritionsource/healthy-eating-plate/

77. Slavin, J. L., & Lloyd, B. (2012). Health Benefits of Fruits and Vegetables. Advances in Nutrition, 3(4), 506–516. https://doi.org/10.3945/an.112.002154

78. Mayo Clinic. (2020, February 8). Men's Health: Tips for aging well. https://www.mayoclinic.org/healthy-lifestyle/mens-health/in-depth/mens-health/art-20047764

79. Wu, G. (2016). Dietary protein intake and human health. Food & Function, 7(3), 1251-1265. https://doi.org/10.1039/C5FO01530H

80. Aune, D., Keum, N., Giovannucci, E., Fadnes, L. T., Boffetta, P., Greenwood, D. C., ... & Norat, T. (2016). Whole grain consumption and risk of cardiovascular disease, cancer, and all cause and cause specific mortality: Systematic review and dose-response meta-analysis of prospective studies. BMJ, 353, i2716. https://doi.org/10.1136/bmj.i2716

81. Aune, D., Giovannucci, E., Boffetta, P., Fadnes, L. T., Keum, N., Norat, T., ... & Tonstad, S. (2017). Fruit and vegetable intake and the risk of cardiovascular disease, total cancer and all-cause mortality—a systematic review and dose-response meta-analysis of prospective studies. International Journal of Epidemiology, 46(3), 1029-1056. https://doi.org/10.1093/ije/dyw319

82. Patterson, R. E., & Sears, D. D. (2017). Metabolic Effects of Intermittent Fasting. Annual Review of Nutrition, 37, 371-393. https://doi.org/10.1146/annurev-nutr-071816-064634

83. de Cabo, R., & Mattson, M. P. (2019). Effects of Intermittent Fasting on Health, Aging, and Disease. The New England Journal of Medicine, 381(26), 2541-2551. https://doi.org/10.1056/NEJMra1905136

84. Popkin, B. M., D'Anci, K. E., & Rosenberg, I. H. (2010). Water, hydration, and health. Nutrition Reviews, 68(8), 439-458. https://doi.org/10.1111/j.1753-4887.2010.00304.x

85. Warren, J. M., Smith, N., & Ashwell, M. (2017). A structured literature review on the role of mindfulness, mindful eating, and intuitive eating in changing eating behaviours: effectiveness and associated potential mechanisms. Nutrition Research Reviews, 30(2), 272-283. https://doi.org/10.1017/S0954422417000154

86. Warburton, D. E., Nicol, C. W., & Bredin, S. S. (2006). Health benefits of physical activity: the evidence. Canadian Medical Association Journal, 174(6), 801-809. https://doi.org/10.1503/cmaj.051351

87. Garber, C. E., Blissmer, B., Deschenes, M. R., Franklin, B. A., Lamonte, M. J., Lee, I. M., ... & Swain, D. P. (2011). American College of Sports Medicine position stand. Quantity and quality of exercise for developing and maintaining cardiorespiratory, musculoskeletal, and neuromotor fitness in apparently healthy adults: guidance for prescribing exercise. Medicine & Science in Sports & Exercise, 43(7), 1334-1359. https://doi.org/10.1249/MSS.0b013e318213fefb

88. Liu, C. J., & Latham, N. K. (2009). Progressive resistance strength training for improving physical function in older adults. The Cochrane Database of Systematic Reviews, 3, CD002759. https://doi.org/10.1002/14651858.CD002759.pub2

89. Sherrington, C., Whitney, J. C., Lord, S. R., Herbert, R. D., Cumming, R. G., & Close, J. C. T. (2008). Effective exercise for the prevention of falls: systematic review and meta-analysis. Journal of the American Geriatrics Society, 56(12), 2234-2243. https://doi.org/10.1111/j.1532-5415.2008.02014.x

90. American College of Sports Medicine. (2013). ACSM's Guidelines for Exercise Testing and Prescription (9th ed.). Lippincott Williams & Wilkins.

91. Paquette M, Bernard S, Ruel I, Blank DW, Genest J, Baass A. Diabetes is associated with an increased risk of cardiovascular disease in patients with familial hypercholesterolemia. J Clin Lipidol. 2019 Jan-Feb;13(1):123-128. doi: 10.1016/j.jacl.2018.09.008. Epub 2018 Sep 17. PMID: 30318454.

92. Obesity, WHO, Retrieve from https://www.who.int/health-topics/obesity

93. Obesity and Overweight, WHO, Retrieve from https://www.who.int/news-room/fact-sheets/detail/obesity-and-overweight
94. Causes of Obesity, CDC Retrieve from https://www.cdc.gov/obesity/basics/causes.html
95. Cassels S. Overweight in the Pacific: links between foreign dependence, global food trade, and obesity in the Federated States of Micronesia. Global Health. 2006 Jul 11;2:10. doi: 10.1186/1744-8603-2-10. PMID: 16834782; PMCID: PMC1533815.
96. World Health Organization. Obesity and overweight. Available from: https://www.who.int/news-room/fact-sheets/detail/obesity-and-overweight (accessed Oct 20, 2023).
97. Health Effects of Overweight and Obesity, Retrieve from https://www.cdc.gov/healthyweight/effects/index.html
98. The Medical Risks of Obesity, PMC, Retrieve from https://www.ncbi.nlm.nih.gov/pmc/articles/PMC2879283/
99. Health Risks of Overweight & Obesity, NIDDK, Retrieve from https://www.niddk.nih.gov/health-information/weight-management/adult-overweight-obesity/health-risks
100. Health Risks Linked to Obesity, WebMD, Retrieve from https://www.webmd.com/obesity/obesity-health-risks
101. Fast Facts – Obesity-Related Chronic Disease, GWU, Retrieve from https://stop.publichealth.gwu.edu/fast-facts/obesity-related-chronic-disease
102. Obesity Medicine - Which Diseases Are Related to Obesity?, Retrieve from https://obesitymedicine.org/diseases-related-to-obesity/
103. Obesity and Chronic Diseases, UMC, Retrieve from https://www.umc.edu/Research/Centers-and-Institutes/Centers/Mississippi-Center-for-Obesity-Research/Resources/Obesity_and_Chronic_Diseases.html
104. Causes and Consequences of Obesity, WHO, Retrieve from https://www.who.int/news-room/questions-and-answers/item/obesity-health-consequences-of-being-overweight
105. Link Obesity and Mental Health, Retrieve from https://www.ncbi.nlm.nih.gov/pmc/articles/PMC6052856/
106. Eating Disorder, National Institute of Mental Health, Retrieve from https://www.nimh.nih.gov/health/topics/eating-disorders/index.shtml
107. Why People Become Overweight, Harvard Medical School, Retrieve from https://www.health.harvard.edu/staying-healthy/why-people-become-overweight
108. Depression and Anxiety, WebMD, Retrieve from https://www.webmd.com/depression/depression-or-anxiety

109. Binge-eating Disorder, Mayo Clinic, Retrieve from https://www.mayoclinic.org/diseases-conditions/binge-eating-disorder/symptoms-causes/syc-20353627
110. Emotional Toll, Retrieve from https://www.healthychildren.org/English/health-issues/conditions/obesity/Pages/The-Emotional-Toll-of-Obesity.aspx
111. Obesity and Overweight, WHO, Retrieve from https://www.who.int/news-room/fact-sheets/detail/obesity-and-overweight
112. Adult Obesity Prevalence Maps, CDC, Retrieved from https://www.cdc.gov/obesity/data/prevalence-maps.html
113. Diabetes Associations in the Pacific, NIH, Retrieve from https://www.ncbi.nlm.nih.gov/pmc/articles/PMC7953240/
114. Obesity in the FSM, NIH, Retrieve from https://pubmed.ncbi.nlm.nih.gov/16834782/
115. Overweight in the Pacific, NCBI, Retrieve from https://www.ncbi.nlm.nih.gov/pmc/articles/PMC1533815
116. Obesity Charts, Retrieve from https://www.niddk.nih.gov/health-information/health-statistics/overweight-obesity
117. Obesity and NHPI, Retrieve from https://minorityhealth.hhs.gov/obesity-and-native-hawaiianspacific-islanders
118. Erectile Dysfunction, Mayo Clinic, Retrieve from https://www.mayoclinic.org/diseases-conditions/erectile-dysfunction/symptoms-causes/syc-20355776
119. Feldman HA, Goldstein I, Hatzichristou DG, Krane RJ, McKinlay JB. Impotence and its medical and psychosocial correlates: Results of the Massachusetts Male Aging Study. J Urol 1994; 151:54–61.

120. Population-level Prevalence, Scientific Report, Retrieve from https://www.nature.com/articles/s41598-023-39968-9
121. Jorgenson E, Matharu N2, Palmer MR,...Van Den Eeden SK. Genetic variation in the SIM1 locus is associated with erectile dysfunction. NIH external link Proc Natl Acad Sci USA 115: 11018-11023, 2018.
122. Roychoudhury, Shubhadeep, Saptaparna Chakraborty, Arun Paul Choudhury, Anandan Das, Niraj Kumar Jha, Petr Slama, Monika Nath, Peter Massanyi, Janne Ruokolainen, and Kavindra Kumar Kesari. 2021. "Environmental Factors-Induced Oxidative Stress: Hormonal and Molecular Pathway Disruptions in Hypogonadism and Erectile Dysfunction" Antioxidants 10, no. 6: 837. https://doi.org/10.3390/antiox10060837
123. Obesity and Erectile Dysfunction, NIH, Retrieve from https://www.ncbi.nlm.nih.gov/pmc/articles/PMC6479091/
124. Obesity and Cardiovascular Disease, Circulation, Retrieve from https://www.ahajournals.org/doi/full/10.1161/CIR.0000000000000973

125. Erectile Dysfunction, WebMd, Retrieve from https://www.webmd.com/erectile-dysfunction/ed-psychological-causes
126. Sexual Medicine, NIH, Retrieve from https://www.ncbi.nlm.nih.gov/pmc/articles/PMC8766276/
127. The Quality of Life and Economic Burden of Erectile Dysfunction, NIH, Retrieve from https://www.ncbi.nlm.nih.gov/pmc/articles/PMC7901407
128. Erectile Dysfunction, NIDDKD, Retrieve from https://www.niddk.nih.gov/health-information/urologic-diseases/erectile-dysfunction
129. Relationship Between Age And Erectile Dysfunction Diagnosis Or Treatment Using Real-World Observational Data In The United States, NIH, Retrieve from https://www.ncbi.nlm.nih.gov/pmc/articles/PMC5540144/
130. Erectile Dysfunction, Cleveland Clinic, Retrieve from https://my.clevelandclinic.org/health/diseases/10035-erectile-dysfunction
131. Erectile Dysfunction and Diabetes, NIH, Retrieve from https://www.ncbi.nlm.nih.gov/pmc/articles/PMC3731873/
132. What Is Erectile Dysfunction?, Urology Care Foundation, Retrieve from https://www.urologyhealth.org/urology-a-z/e/
133. What Are the Treatment Options For Erectile Dysfunction?, Medical News Today, Retrieve from https://www.medicalnewstoday.com/articles/323688
134. Vascular (Arterial And Venous) Surgery For Erectile Dysfunction, Springer, Retrieve from https://link.springer.com/chapter/10.1007/978-3-030-21447-0_50
135. A Psychosocial Approach to Erectile Dysfunction, NIH, Retrieve from https://www.ncbi.nlm.nih.gov/pmc/articles/PMC8766276/
136. Shoag JE, Mittal S, Hu JC. Reevaluating PSA testing rates in the PLCO trial. N Engl J Med. 2016;374(18):1795-1796.
137. Shoag JE, Nyame YA, Gulati R, Etzioni R, Hu JC. Reconsidering the trade-offs of prostate cancer screening. N Engl J Med. 2020;382(25):2465-2468.
138. Bryant AK, Lee KM, Alba PR, et al. Association of prostate-specific antigen screening rates with subsequent metastatic prostate cancer incidence at US Veterans Health Administration facilities. JAMA Oncol. 2022;8(12):1747-1755.
139. Légaré F, Ratte S, Gravel K, Graham ID. Barriers and facilitators to implementing shared decision-making in clinical practice: update of a systematic review of health professionals' perceptions. Patient Educ Couns. 2008;73(3):526-535.
140. Jiang C, Fedewa SA, Wen Y, Jemal A, Han X. Shared decision making and prostate-specific antigen based prostate cancer screening following the 2018 update of USPSTF screening guideline. Prostate Cancer Prostatic Dis. 2021;24(1):77-80.
141. Donovan JL, Hamdy FC, Lane JA, et al. Patient-reported outcomes after monitoring, surgery, or radiotherapy for prostate cancer. N Engl J Med. 2016;375(15):1425-1437.

142. Donovan JL, Hamdy FC, Lane JA, et al. Patient-reported outcomes 12 years after localized prostate cancer treatment. NEJM Evid. 2023;10.1056/EVIDoa2300018.
143. (1993) Mental Illness in Micronesia, MicSem Publications, Retrieved from: https://micsem.org/micronesian-counselo/mental-illness-in-micronesia/
144. The Power of Zero, David McKnight. Retrieved from https://www.youtube.com/watch?v=NmbJiAILGLc

Request for Review

Dear Reader,

Hi there! We wanted to reach out personally and have a heartfelt chat with you. We hope you're doing great and embracing the joys of life!

Before we dive in, we want to take a moment to express our heartfelt gratitude for selecting *The Age of Optimal Health: A Comprehensive Guide for Men Over 50 to Maintain an Active Lifestyle, Ensure Proper Nutrition, and Take Preventative Measures* by Surleigh Tara. We can't thank you enough for investing your valuable time in our book and placing your trust in us.

As authors and publishers, we pour our hearts and souls into creating content that speaks directly to individuals like you. We firmly believe that every person's perspective is unique and incredibly valuable. That's why we're reaching out to you today – to kindly ask for your support in sharing your personal thoughts and experiences by writing a review.

Your review holds incredible power. It has the ability to touch the lives of other men over 50 who are on a similar journey toward guidance, inspiration, and a more fulfilling life. By sharing your own personal journey, insights, and reflections, you become a beacon of light for others.

We encourage you to craft a review that is deeply personal, filled with your unique experiences and the profound impact the book has had on you. Here are a few prompts to help you gather your thoughts:

1. How has *The Age of Optimal Health* resonated with your own path as a man over 50? Can you share your specific challenges and how the book has provided practical solutions and insightful perspectives?

2. Have specific recommendations or strategies from the book positively influenced your lifestyle, nutrition choices, or preventative measures? How have these changes affected your overall well-being?

3. As authors and publishers, we have poured our hearts into this book. Surleigh Tara has gone the extra mile by sharing his wisdom and knowledge. Has his writing style captivated your attention and made the content relatable and easily digestible? Are there any personal stories or anecdotes that have left a lasting impression on you?

4. Imagine you're speaking to a dear friend who hasn't had the opportunity to read the book. What key message would you want to convey about its value and the impact it has had on your life?

Your honest and heartfelt review will not only provide invaluable feedback to the author but also serve as a guiding light for others seeking positive transformations. Your words possess the power to inspire and lead others toward a healthier and more fulfilling life.

Thank you for considering sharing your unique and honest

review and for being an inspiration to others.

With deep appreciation,

Surleigh Tara.

www.ingramcontent.com/pod-product-compliance
Lightning Source LLC
Chambersburg PA
CBHW022045020426
42335CB00012B/552